cooking
without
Made easy

recipes free from added
gluten, sugar, yeast
and dairy produce

barbara cousins

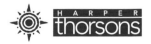

HARPER thorsons

HarperThorsons
An Imprint of HarperCollins*Publishers*
77–85 Fulham Palace Road,
Hammersmith, London W6 8JB

The website address is: www.thorsonselement.com

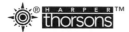

and *HarperThorsons* are trademarks of
HarperCollins*Publishers* Ltd

First published by HarperThorsons 2005

10 9 8 7

© Barbara Cousins 2005

Barbara Cousins asserts the moral right to
be identified as the author of this work

A catalogue record of this book
is available from the British Library

ISBN-13   978-0-00-719876-4
ISBN-10   0-00-719876-0

Printed and bound in Great Britain by
Martins the Printers Ltd, Berwick upon Tweed

Contents

The cure of the part should not be attempted without treatment of the whole. No attempt should be made to cure the body without the soul, if the head and body are to be healthy, you must begin by curing the mind … for this is the great error of our day in the treatment of the human body, that physicians first separate the soul from the body.

Plato, in the fifth century BC

Introduction

Having spent the last 18 years in practice as a nutritional therapist, I felt I needed to write this third book in the *Cooking Without* series to summarize the knowledge I have acquired during this time. I also wanted to include lots of easy recipes because, having learnt during the last 18 years to be much kinder to myself, I like to cook dishes that are uncomplicated as well as healthy.

My first book, *Cooking Without*, came as a result of clients asking for recipes because they didn't know how to cook without wheat, sugar, yeast and dairy produce. When my self-published version was eventually taken over by Thorsons I added a section about detoxification so that the book could be used as a do it-yourself manual by anyone wishing to put the regime into practice and improve their health. Next came *Vegetarian Cooking Without*, which has a section covering various health problems and the insights that I have gained over the years through dealing with my own health as well as that of my clients.

This book feels like the final one of a trilogy. It is a summary of the effect that 'cooking without' can have on peoples' lives. In it I have used my own story, and those of some of my clients, to help explain the remarkable changes that can happen when detoxification takes place. It has always been my aim not only to alleviate the physical symptoms of my clients, but

> In all the case histories quoted in this book the names and precise circumstances of individuals have been changed in order to protect their privacy.

to uncover the reasons why they became ill. Physical symptoms are just the body trying to talk to us, to encourage us to look below the surface and find the answers.

We need to reach a point where we can be in the moment rather than in the past or future, where we can let go of control and have trust and faith, where we can be in touch with our intuition rather than in our heads – a place where health replaces disease. This is what *Cooking Without Made Easy* and my other two books are about. It is, I believe, the work I came here to do and to pass on to others.

Where it all began

My interest in diet and nutrition really took off after the birth of my first son in 1974. Three weeks after my son was born he developed a throat infection. His birth had been long and difficult and I had accepted all the pain relief I was offered. I'm now sure that his first infection was his body's way of throwing off the toxicity from the drugs that he too must have ingested. When the doctor gave him his first antibiotic I had an instinctive feeling that this was not the right thing to do. A month later he went down with another infection. His little body had overcome the suppression of the antibiotic and was now trying to eliminate the previous toxicity, along with that of the antibiotic.

Fortunately, there was a health food shop in the town where I lived and although in those days the supplements available were limited, it was suggested that I try vitamin C. It did the trick. When infections did occur over the years I always went to the doctor for a diagnosis, but he soon learned that I preferred not to use drugs. Sometimes I went away with a prescription just in case, but I always followed a visit to the doctor with one to the health food shop, and so my son avoided the antibiotic treadmill.

When my second son was born 18 months later, my own health began to suffer. For the first time in my life I was lacking in energy and my skin and hair felt lifeless. This spurred me on to examine and improve our diet. I started baking wholemeal bread, cut down on sugar and included more fruit and vegetables in the family diet. My health improved rapidly, my children blossomed and as a result I became a convert to healthy eating.

Healing physical symptoms

In the early days my use of nutrition was aimed at – and succeeded in – eliminating physical symptoms. Over the years, many of my clients have seen the dramatic effect that a change of diet can have on their physical health. Often, after only a few weeks on a new regime, the change is remarkable and many struggle to believe that diet can be so powerful. This was the situation in the following three case histories.

David

David came to me because he was suffering from anxiety symptoms. He was waking in the night feeling anxious, frightened and panicky, and had palpitations. During the day he was tired, couldn't concentrate and often felt depressed, irritable and full of irrational fears. Three weeks after the start of a 'cooking without' dietary regime David was delighted with his improvement. He was less anxious, less tired and had had only one anxiety attack in the night. He continued to make improvements, becoming much calmer and less prone to mood swings. His concentration improved and life took on new meaning. David's problems stemmed from an allergy that was causing his blood sugar to drop. However, once the problem foods were removed from his diet and his blood sugar was supported with the right kind of food at regular intervals, his problems ceased.

Gail

Gail had been suffering from arthritis for 15 years and migraines for 20 years when she came for a consultation. Within just three weeks she experienced an improvement – she had more energy, no headaches and fewer aches and pains. Six weeks later she was feeling really well and, for the first time in years, her periods were on time. Gail continued to visit me over the years whenever she had a problem and although she did have a little residual damage in her feet from the arthritis, her original problems did not recur.

Gail was a teacher and had spent years living on her adrenalin, taking more out of her body than she was putting back in. Once on a nutritionally-sound programme, her body was able to eliminate some of the backlog of toxicity that was at the root of her problems.

Kirsty tells her story

'When I first began seeing Barbara, I was feeling tired, bloated and constipated, and I had been putting weight on steadily for five years. I had gradually become anaemic and was at a loss as to why this was happening, as I had not altered my diet or lifestyle. After overcoming the shock of such a drastic change in diet – I had to eat six times a day and a minimum amount – I started to feel better and found I had more energy and was calmer and more relaxed.

But the biggest change came when I cut out all dairy produce (an allergy test had proved that I was intolerant to dairy from any animal). I stopped having digestive rumblings, wind and constipation, and my sinuses cleared up. I also started losing weight – 30kg in a year, which translates to 1lb per week, a healthy rate. I have not needed to see Barbara for some time now, but I still keep pretty much to her diet.

Detective work

Although over the years most clients have seen some improvements in their health by their second appointment, not everyone experiences overnight success. Nutritional therapy is a little like detective work – it involves looking for signs that the body produces, in order to diagnose and prescribe, and then watching how the body reacts to any changes. Most clients have a few ups and downs, as we untangle the causes of their problems, before they eventually settle on the road to recovery.

Bernice

Bernice had ulcerative colitis, which caused cramping pains and urgent visits to the loo with the passing of blood and mucus. She was tired all the time and depressed because of her ill health. By her second visit she had much more energy, she was less depressed and the ache in her colon had disappeared. Bernice was enjoying feeling much better so she made the most of it and started catching up on all the jobs she had left undone. Unfortunately, her health soon began to deteriorate again. At this stage in her recovery there simply wasn't enough energy available for healing and catching up. But at least Bernice was learning. Her next lesson, once she had improved still further and started venturing out into society again, was how important it is to stay with the diet. She was feeling better and starting to enjoy life, so the diet slipped – as did her health. We had another year of ups and downs as Bernice adjusted to her new regime but now at least she has an answer to her problems.

Sarah

Sarah was quite poorly when she first came to see me. She had serious diges-tive problems, which included severe pain, bloating and constipation, as well as very poor energy levels, and thrush. It was obvious that Sarah had intolerances to several foods and although coming off these produced a slight improvement in her health, we had a long way to go. Over the course of a few years, Sarah and I learned a lot about her body as we untangled the web of clues that her illness threw up. Sarah's body was so finely balanced that any major change caused a reaction, therefore we had to proceed very slowly.

We discovered that Sarah's liver was struggling to cope. When it was happy the severe pains she had in her shoulder disappeared; when it wasn't happy the food she ate just sat in her stomach. We learned that foods with a warming energy (I talk about the energetics of foods in Vegetarian Cooking Without) *helped her digestion, while too many foods with a cold energy shut it down. In fact, Sarah became so good at knowing the energy of foods because of her body's reaction to them that, in the end, she was teaching me. We learned that too much protein overloaded her digestion, but equally too much carbohydrate or vegetables and she had a reaction. We tried the 'Hay diet' and the 'Eat right for your type' diet but in the end we had no option but to follow the diet that Sarah's body was determining and, as a result, her health improved.*

Body, mind and spirit

In all the above case histories the individuals were able to alleviate their symptoms – but only if they followed the diet. However, what started to interest me as far back as the 1970s were the reasons behind why people became ill. In those days, as well as reading all I could find on nutrition, I studied astrology, spiritual healing, Bach flower remedies, yoga and anything else I could find on holistic health. The link between body, mind and spirit was starting to become clear. Over the years, however, not all my clients have been ready to delve deeper and look at the reasons behind why they became ill. Many just wanted their physical symptoms to disappear so that they could carry on with their lives. While it is not up to me to decide when the time is right for anyone to delve deeper, I was often responsible for giving people the odd nudge, which sometimes did and sometimes didn't make them think.

When ready to consider the deeper reasons for their illness, clients come into the consultation room and instead of talking about their physical problems, will say things like 'I've been thinking'. Suddenly their physical health, which was their priority, is no longer paramount and their desire for a greater understanding takes precedence. I'm always thrilled when this happens because it means that we can move on to a deeper level of detoxification. Eventually, when their mental and emotional bodies are satisfied, they come into the consultation room saying things like 'Why am I here?' or 'Do you believe in a higher power?' At this point it's time to move on to the next stage – the spiritual. This progression never ceases to amaze and delight me and I'm forever in debt to all the clients who have allowed me to be part of their journeys and taught me so much along the way. But it also makes me so aware of how much society's loss of spirituality is in direct proportion to its dietary decline.

Detoxification

Having originally trained as a home economist, I eventually retrained as a nutritional therapist in the mid eighties. During my training I began to learn the principles of detoxification, which involves using strict dietary principles (as outlined in *Cooking Without*) and supplementation to assist the body to eliminate toxicity. It was this training that made me realize that nutrition can be used as a catalyst for detoxifying the body on various levels. Once the physical body starts to heal, detoxification moves on to a mental and emotional level, and finally reveals a spiritual body hidden beneath.

Once I started to detoxify I started on a journey of self-discovery. As well as improving my physical health, I started to uncover the real me that had been buried beneath the layers of ideas and conditioning that I had taken on board from others over the years. It was like peeling off the layers of an onion. The more dysfunctional our past, the more layers we develop in order to cope and protect ourselves. These layers build up from early childhood and directly influence our view of the world.

Developing layers

As babies, we come into this world with nothing in our heads but a strong intuitive drive to meet our needs and be true to ourselves. Watch a little child playing. One minute it is totally engrossed then suddenly it has had enough and moves on to something else or comes for a hug or a drink. If a child were allowed to grow up keeping in touch with its intuition then as an adult it would build up far fewer layers. Unfortunately, children are continually being told to use their heads and not their hearts, 'finish your maths before you go out to play'. Some of this is necessary, of course – our heads tell us to look both ways before crossing the road or not to eat food that is too hot. However, living too much in our heads means that we lose touch with our sense of self. As always in life, the art is in finding a balance. Here I am talking about healthy children in good homes, but imagine the damage that can be inflicted through neglect or physical and mental abuse.

Losing our sense of self means that we are being, doing and thinking what others have taught us. Detoxification is about stripping off the layers and uncovering our core self, which is always a beautiful expression of our soul. I believe that one of the things we are all here to do is to peel off the layers in order to reach our intuition and true potential, and hence follow the path our soul chose.

Soul paths

I think that we all come into this world with the potential to be something special. I don't mean famous or rich, but with a potential to be a good mother, a special friend, a great teacher ... It's as though our souls decide before we are born and they know what we are meant to do – but, when we are born, no one lets us in on the arrangement. However, if we can learn to trust a higher power and be in touch with our intuition, then the universe can guide us along the path we are meant to tread. There will still be difficulties along the way, as these are necessary in order for us to grow, but it's when we rely on our heads and want to be in control that we create the most problems. When we flow with life and are open, the universe guides us gently forward, creating synchronicities and coincidences. Opportunities and directions appear and we know – rather than think – that we are doing the right thing.

Uncovering our life path
There are many ways of uncovering our intuition, the real us and our life path, and each individual must choose the right way for themselves. Everything that we need to know is inside us and we must find a way of going inside to find that information. What is right for me and what is my truth may not be yours. It's as though we are all little spiders heading back to a higher consciousness on our own little threads. I cannot jump onto your thread and you cannot jump onto mine. Our intuition is the higher consciousness talking to us, so the ideas contained in this or any other book should only be considered right for you if they resonate with your truth.

The method I found of uncovering the real me, and the way I've used to help my clients find their truth, has been through diet and detoxification. The only way that I can know that an individual is better is when they have uncovered the reasons why they became ill and have found their path in life.

Julie

Julie came to me after an operation for cancer. The cancer was a wake-up call and Julie knew that she had to change if she was to survive. However, she didn't know what changes she needed to make and the thought of making any filled her with fear. Julie embarked on a serious detoxification regime that, day by day, led her to new insights about herself and her lifestyle. She had a mundane office job that was way below her capabilities, but it enabled her to act as a support system for her husband and family. I remember Julie on her first visit: she had her blonde hair swept up in a very eighties' style and was dressed in a flimsy suit and camisole on a cold winter's day. I wanted to wrap her up in a warm sweater and jeans, but the image she portrayed was the one her husband liked – the feminine woman who needed him, was there for him and who didn't rock the boat.

As Julie progressed she started to read alternative books, make new friends and became vegetarian. She studied counselling at nightschool and although she wanted her husband to be part of her new life, he was clearly not impressed because she wasn't always there at his beck and call.

Julie blossomed and grew stronger as the months passed. Eventually the inevitable happened and she left her husband. She was willing to stay, but only if her husband was prepared to accept the person she was – but alas, he wasn't. He wanted life to go back to the way it had been because that meant he didn't have to face his own issues (Julie had always rescued him from these). Leaving was very tough for Julie, as she had to face many fears. Would she be able to support herself? Would she be able to stand up for herself and cope with the running of a home on her own? Would the children understand why she was doing this?

Julie not only survived, but went from strength to strength. She finished her counselling course and was asked to go back and do some teaching. She set up a private practice and became very successful – and guess what? She changed her hairstyle and threw away the flimsy suits.

Maralyn tells her story
'I had suffered from bouts of depression for 30 years when I went to see Barbara. During these times I was incapable of work and lost interest in everyone and everything. I had tried all the usual antidepressant drugs and had seen psychiatrists and psychologists, but nothing seemed to help.

Initially, Barbara reviewed my diet and explained that with intolerances (I had become aware that I was intolerant to yeast) a restricted diet was important but until the emotions were dealt with, the allergy would not resolve itself. Through detoxification, vitamin and mineral supplements and dealing with my emotions relating to a very unhappy, restricted childhood, I slowly started to feel much better.

I can honestly say that since meeting Barbara I have never suffered a repeat bout of depression. That was over five years ago and now I really understand the saying 'We are what we eat'.

Looking back at my own childhood

I was the second of two children, with a brother two years older. We grew up on an isolated farm and my parents worked very hard, so they had little time for looking after children. My father was moody, heading towards manic depression and locked in his own inner world of torment. He had lost his mother when very young and had had a tough upbringing. I soon learnt that it was best not to have any needs if I wanted to please my parents and, as a result, I began to cut off from my emotions at an early age. I learnt to smile rather than cry, even though I was hurting inside. I also learnt that if I did something exceptional I received some attention – and so I became a people pleaser and an over-achiever. I started losing touch with my intuition by spending time in my head trying to be what everyone wanted me to be and assuming that I was the cause of any deficit. Not surprisingly, this resulted in an unrealistically negative self-image, which laid the foundations for a life that would need many knocks to get me to examine, and begin to peel off, the layers I had developed through childhood and beyond.

Being in touch with our true selves and our intuition doesn't prevent us from making mistakes, but it helps us recognize when we've made them, because things don't feel right. I had stopped feeling, therefore it was very difficult to distinguish between what felt right and wrong.

Logic versus intuition

When I talk about being 'in our heads', I'm talking about using the left side of the brain, which is the logical side. This logical side works things out by analysing the criteria rather than by assessing how things feel. In contrast, our intuition whispers to us between our thoughts. When we go with our intuition we are using the right side of our brain and we feel comfortable with what we are doing. Frequently, when clients are trying to work out what job they would like to do, they make the mistake of trying to work it out by analysing what they are good at. They may think they are good at maths and so start looking at jobs where they could use this skill, such as accountancy or teaching. However, it's more important to look for something that feeds the soul – if it doesn't, it can become soul-destroying. We won't ever reach our full potential in life or be really happy if we don't follow our hearts. I believe that when we find our true path in life, our job will feel more like a hobby. When I discovered nutritional therapy I simply wanted to read and learn everything I could about the subject. It was a natural extension to turn it into a job.

Helen tells her story of a change in direction

'I had a high-profile job in marketing when I first went to see Barbara. I was travelling the country, working long hours, and although I earned a good salary, most of it was spent sustaining my working lifestyle. By the time I reached 31 I had undergone four operations to remove endometriosis, but it always came back. I turned to nutritional therapy out of sheer desperation. Within three weeks I was looking and feeling much better. I wasn't putting in the same hours in the office because I needed time to shop and cook, but the work I produced reflected a new clarity and confidence. Even my boss commented on it.

Over the next few years I made some major changes in my life. I let go of the security and trappings of my career and left to set up a consultancy. As I downsized I realized that the freedom and satisfaction I now felt easily replaced the big salary and company car. Creating more space in my life meant that I had time to walk, horse ride and spend more time with nature and the people who mattered to me. I felt much more in touch with myself as I began to live more from my heart than from my head.

My next major change came when I took off with my partner on a 16-month, round-the-world trip. That really was a leap of faith, to let go of everything and just trust. It turned out to be the most amazing time of my life. While travelling I started to write a travelogue, tapping into a creativity that had lain dormant since my schooldays. Now I am working on this material and hope in the future to become a travel writer. Combining travel and writing would be my dream way of life. And the endometriosis? It just disappeared, much to my consultant's surprise. I am so glad that I took those first steps towards controlling my own health and my life.'

Detoxification is like a life jigsaw

When I look back at the person I was before I started to detoxify I can hardly believe that I'm the same person. Unfortunately, that doesn't mean that 'I've arrived', as I'm constantly gaining new insights and growing stronger, and will continue to do so until the day I die. But looking back lets me see how eating the right food has enabled me to recognize the next stage in my development; to see issues that needed working on as they appeared and then, after working through these, moving on again, rather than staying stuck and repeating the same mistakes.

I often liken detoxification to a life jigsaw. It's as though a jigsaw has been put together but the pieces are not all in the right places. When you start to detoxify it's as if someone has thrown your life's jigsaw onto the floor and it has smashed into hundreds of pieces. It is then up to you to fit it back together – only this time with all the pieces in their right places. At first this is difficult because you know that your life doesn't work but you haven't a clue what the jigsaw is meant to look like. At this point you need a certain amount of trust and faith that your new direction will appear. And it does.

You find yourself considering a piece of the jigsaw that holds the key to a certain area of your life. It may be a piece about guilt, or pleasing people and you spend a few days or weeks thinking about how this affects your life and how you could change it. Then one day you consider another jigsaw piece and have a new insightful realization, and suddenly you've fitted two pieces of the jigsaw together. And so it goes on; as you peel the layers from yourself you gradually build up a new picture of the real you. I'm still working on my jigsaw; I still have issues with lack of self-worth but the universe keeps providing me with opportunities to grow.

My lack of self-worth

My parents were basically good people who loved me in their own way, and they were doing what they thought was their best. However, their attitudes to parenting were based on their own dysfunctional upbringings. They were very money orientated – to them, money in the bank equalled security. I had very few toys or books, the most basic of clothes and the home didn't contain any of life's luxuries. I remember birthdays and Christmases with nothing to open – instead my parents put money in a bank account for when we were older. We never had a Christmas tree or bedtime stories; I didn't go on holiday or have friends to stay. The message that I constantly received as a child was that I didn't matter but money did. Self-worth was one of the lessons my soul obviously came here to learn.

Wanting the perfect marriage

My lack of self-worth and inability to be in touch with my feelings have drawn many lessons to me throughout my life. Because of my relationship with my father, I was attracted to emotionally unavailable men, whom I hoped would fulfil my every need if I loved them enough. Basically, there was still a little girl inside of me desperately wanting the love of her father, so I transferred this on to the men in my life. My husband had come from an equally cold and dysfunctional family, where he was taught fear and learnt to control in order to allay his fears. Once married, I also gained an equally controlling mother-in-law and so my self-worth took another battering and my 'people pleaser' ran on overdrive. I wanted to have the perfect marriage and I was willing to suppress any discomfort I felt in order to make this happen. I loved being married and I loved being a mum to my two boys. I went to no end of trouble to make the home a warm, comfortable environment and was determined to make sure my children felt loved and secure. But I also felt trapped and controlled. No one was interested in how I felt and whether my needs were being met and I didn't have sufficient self-worth to put my case forward. If I did try to assert myself then I tapped into my husband's fears, and he couldn't cope, so I suppressed my feelings yet again. And, of course, I never dreamt of talking to anyone outside the home, as my sense of self-worth was invested in being perfect.

Eventually I was introduced to astrology and I started to question what life was about. I read alternative books and looked at what was going on in my life from a different perspective. The floodgates of emotion eventually burst when my dog was accidentally killed. I remember finding her and wanting to cry but not being able to at first – but when I did start crying, I couldn't stop. I wasn't just crying for her, devastated though I was, I was crying for me and all the hurts and injustices I'd suffered throughout my life and had never cried about before. That marked a turning point in my life. I could no longer be what everyone else wanted me to be; I had to start standing up for what I needed.

It was hard, however, to put the blinkers on and follow the path that was revealing itself to me. I felt like I was on a long, straight road that disappears into the horizon. On each side the land was lower than the road and all along were people trying to pull me off my path and divert me. It would have been easy for me to use everyone else as an excuse for not following my own star, especially as I didn't know where my star was taking me. We are, however, always aware of the next step and the rest is revealed to us one day at a time.

Facing the fear

When I eventually re-trained and set up a healing clinic in the mid-eighties I was full of fear. Alternative medicine wasn't exactly popular in Manchester, and nutrition was at the bottom of the list. I was fearful of failure, of not being able to help people, or being thought of as foolish. But more than that, I was frightened of putting myself, and my growth, first.

Self-growth, however, is like giving birth – you can't stop it once it's started, and so I kept moving forward and taking the next step. I was facing the fear and doing it anyway.

I also learnt to trust in God and the universe. For God is like a kind, caring father, who's going to push a little so that we grow, but he will never put us in situations where we really can't cope. And so my clinic was a success. The more I trusted God and handed over control, the more he helped. I was frequently guided to treatments or found myself uttering statements that I didn't know I knew.

Natalie

Natalie was a client of mine who had three young children and a husband. She was organized, hard working and capable, with a tremendous amount of untapped potential. She wanted to set up her own business, but she had a husband who was married to his job. This meant that he arrived home later than he said he would, ended up working weekends or on his days off and, when he was around, his mind was elsewhere rather than on his family. Natalie took responsibility for everything concerning the home and family. In their early married life, when the children were young, Natalie didn't mind too much; it was only when the children started school that she resented being the support system with no hope of a career of her own. But Natalie avoided facing the fear involved in forcing the necessary changes – instead she used food as a substitute for love and to cover up any feelings of discomfort.

Eventually, Natalie came to see me when she developed arthritis. She went home from her first consultation enthusiastic about the slender, healthy body that she felt she would soon regain. A few months later she was back in my consulting room saying that she was going to have to give up on the treatment. She was having a few problems with her husband and needed time to sort these out before she resumed treatment. It seems that Natalie had started expressing how she felt as she had started to detoxify and this had caused problems between her and her husband. I tried to explain that this was all part of the detoxification, that health wasn't just about being slim and fit but about being true to our selves and in touch with our own potential and power. It's not an easy concept to grasp and Natalie didn't even want to try. Things were very uncomfortable and she didn't like it, so she chose to go back to her old way of life rather than rock the boat. She took menial jobs that fitted in with the children's schooling and holidays and continued to have health problems. Natalie chose to remain toxic rather than face and move through her pain.

Learning to love ourselves

If we are not following our true path and meeting our needs, then we are not loving and caring for ourselves. We then need other people or other things to serve as a substitute for love, and to use as an anaesthetic to cover up our basic unease. Natalie used food, but whatever 'substance' you are addicted to – be it alcohol, drugs, sex, television, shopping or gambling – you are using something or someone to cover up your pain. Natalie's husband used work. I used sweet food, but I also always wanted other people to love me because I didn't love myself. I always dreamt of wonderful birthdays and Christmases when I would be showered with gifts. I always hoped that my husband would buy me chocolates and flowers and book tables in romantic candlelit restaurants, but it never happened. And it didn't happen because the universe wanted me to learn to love myself. This lesson repeated itself so many times in my life that I eventually wrote the following quote, which I've handed out regularly to clients over the years: 'We don't get what we want in life, we get what we need in order to grow. When we've grown we get what we've always wanted, only then we don't need it any more'.

The more I wanted others to show how much they loved me, the less love I received. Eventually, however, when I started loving myself sufficiently, others started treating me better, but guess what? I didn't need it any more. That doesn't mean that I didn't appreciate their kindness, because I did, but it became a bonus and an indulgence rather than a necessity.

Learning to love ourselves doesn't make relationships redundant, but it does mean that we move on from dysfunctional relationships where we are too dependent on our partners to meet our needs, to a relationship where two people come together for mutual growth and benefit, one in which each is able to stand on their own feet, meet their needs and follow their own path.

Being human

During the time I was learning to love myself I suddenly found myself attracted to someone new. The feeling was mutual and I was shocked. I thought I had the perfect marriage, so what was happening? However, in reality I was more in touch with what I imagined my marriage to be, rather than the real thing. Looking back, I did the best possible thing – I told my husband what was happening and how I was feeling. This opened up a level of communication we'd never had before, enabling us both to face issues, many of which we'd not even known were there. These issues were ones that would have come up in the new relationship, if I'd chosen to move on, because like attracts like. I was attracting someone who would have been there to teach me in the same way that my husband was. The only time a new relationship is necessary is when an old one is over; when one partner has moved on and grown and the other hasn't and doesn't want to.

I'd not been in touch enough with my feelings to be able to be honest with myself, and now suddenly feelings were overwhelming me. I had always tried to be 'Miss Perfect', using perfectionism and super-achievement as a shield to cover up for my lack of self-worth. But suddenly I felt very human, and human beings are not infallible. It was actually a relief to realize that I was human; that I wasn't perfect and that it was actually all right not to be. I was being taught to love myself, warts and all. Even though I hadn't consciously attracted someone else, I'd obviously done so unconsciously. Inside of me there was still that little girl who just wanted to be loved and who felt better about herself knowing that others loved her. It made me much more aware of the work I still needed to do in order to love myself sufficiently so that I wasn't so needy. I had to be able to stand on my own two feet, whoever I was with.

My husband's fear of losing me made him face up to the fears that had prevented him from wanting to listen to my problems in the past. If I wasn't happy he felt vulnerable, inadequate and lacking in control. In turn, I sensed his pain and tapped into my own fears of losing him, because I wasn't making him happy, therefore I'd always suppressed my feelings and backed down. Now that things were changing, I was able to tell him about all the occasions when I'd been unhappy, when I'd felt unsupported, when I'd been very hurt. I cried and I got angry. Finally being honest with each other allowed us both to grow and we became closer – and more open with each other than we'd ever been.

Jane's story

Jane was a client of mine. She was married with two boys and had what she considered a good marriage. Jane was a carer – she loved looking after her home and family and never complained. Her husband had his own business and worked long hours, but he was a good father and always found time for the boys. He would take them to football matches or play with them on the computer and had built up a good relationship with his sons. However, the family didn't do many things together – they rarely went out for the day, or to the seaside or even on holiday. Jane would often entertain her husband's work colleagues, despite the fact that she didn't like some of them. She also did the book keeping for the business because it helped out and saved the company money, rather than because she enjoyed it.

Jane had started taking antidepressants in order to cope with her father's long illness and subsequent death. The drugs helped her to suppress the emotions she needed to work through, many of which stemmed from the lack of support she was receiving. She came to me to help her come off the antidepressant. However, each time she cut down the amount she was taking she became anxious. This was caused by mental and emotional toxicity that she needed to work through and leave behind. Irrational feelings make sense when we understand what's behind them, therefore I suggested that she came regularly for support in order to begin to work through the issues at the root of her anxiety. Unfortunately, this never happened as Jane always managed to cancel her next appointment before we'd done any constructive work. In her heart, though, Jane knew that this was the right way forward and would arrive back in my consulting room six months down the line, back on the full amount of antidepressants. We'd then start the process again, only for her to give up yet again.

Eventually, the drugs were not sufficient and Jane started to turn to alcohol. She enjoyed a glass of wine and considered it a treat, but what had been an occasional tipple became a daily necessity, something that she turned to whenever she felt anxious, uncomfortable, unloved or put upon. As a result, the emotions that were trying to come to the surface were suppressed yet again.

Then one day Jane met someone else, had an affair and moved out of the family home. Everyone was shocked, including Jane. She couldn't understand what was happening to her; what this compulsion was that was dragging her away from what she thought was a good marriage. She said that she hadn't minded always being there and looking after everyone, yet the man she had met was giving her all the things that she'd never had in her marriage: weekends away, days out, holidays, fun, time for her, and support. Jane had used *drugs and alcohol over the years to suppress the real her. She had tapped into one side of her personality, the carer, but had ignored a part of her soul that was crying out for attention.*

Unfortunately, the story doesn't have a happy ending. Eventually, Jane's husband took the opportunity to move to America and the boys decided to go with him. They never forgave their mother for breaking up their home. And so Jane gained and lost a great deal.

It's not for me to judge if Jane did the right thing. Only her soul knows if she is on the right path, but I can't help wondering what would have happened if Jane had been able to stay with the diet and detoxification.

The last few case histories have been about women getting in touch with their feelings and having sufficient power to act upon them, but I haven't yet talked about men. At present, the world is going through a great metamorphosis and this is affecting men as well as women. In the past, women were seen as nurturers and men as achievers. Now this is changing and the change is causing a lot of confusion, pain and loneliness. Men and women are becoming more androgynous and becoming whole within themselves – sometimes receptive, sometimes assertive. Relationships between men and women are changing to one of mutual understanding, companionship and growth. We are learning to talk to each other as equals and human beings instead of trying to fit into stereotypical male and female roles.

The patriarchal domination of the world is hopefully coming to an end. The feminine represents the kind of power we need in order to overcome the warmongering, empire-building greed that is bringing our planet to the edge of extinction. The fear and disrespect of the feminine emerges from a fear and distrust of one's own feelings. There is no room in a male-dominated system for them. If one really felt the effects of one's actions – whether the act is suppressing a race, abusing a child or allowing starvation to occur –

most people could not continue to live with the internal conflict it would cause.

Fortunately, many men today are starting to become aware of their feminine side and are more ready to show their feelings. They are letting go of control and starting to respond from their hearts. They are learning to tap into a higher spiritual power and flow with their intuition.

Jonathan's story

Jonathan's childhood was characterized by the dominance of his strict father, who wanted Jonathan to be 'a success in life'. Being a very sensitive and caring child who loved animals and art, Jonathan did not fit in well with the role he was being forced to play. When Jonathan arrived home from school, he wasn't allowed to play with his friends, watch television or draw. If he didn't have homework from school, his dad set some for him to do. He was forced to play rugby and take part in judo, even though he hated these contact sports. He was, however, quite a good long-distance runner, but instead of being able to enjoy his talent his father killed his enthusiasm. Jonathan told me about a time when he was leading a race but ran out of stamina and was overtaken in the last leg. He was runner-up in the race, but his father was furious that he had allowed himself to be overtaken.

Jonathan was only in his early twenties and at university when he had a nervous breakdown. He was doing all the things he thought he was meant to do in order to enjoy life, such as going to football matches with his friends and for drinking sessions at the pub, but inside he was empty and unhappy and he didn't know why.

Jonathan came to me because he instinctively knew that the drugs he had been given for his breakdown were only masking the symptoms. He didn't know what to expect, or even if I could help him, but he knew that there had to be another way. He happily changed his diet and started to detoxify. He was so thrilled that someone understood what he was going through and was offering him a way out of his trauma. As Jonathan detoxified he was able to work through some of the issues in his past, though now he was able to see what went on from a more mature perspective.

Jonathan still spoke to his father regularly but he hated their phone calls or meetings because his father still tried to tell him what to do. A real breakthrough occurred when Jonathan stood up for himself one day and told his father what HE thought and what HE was going to do. His father refused to speak to him for quite a few weeks but Jonathan didn't back down. He also worked through the anger he felt towards his mother for not sticking up for him when he was a child. Eventually, Jonathan was able to build up a relationship with both his parents. It was never going to be easy because his parents hadn't moved on and Jonathan had. However, he was able to accept them for what they were – and even forgive them for the past – and carry on to complete for himself the job of parenting.

Jonathan started to develop a strong psychic talent as he tapped into his feminine side. I'm not sure where this will take him, as he is still young, but he is now open to whatever the universe has in mind. It hasn't been an easy path for him and he has suffered great pain and loneliness along the way. The things that are important to him now do not fit in with his old lifestyle – or that of the youth culture of today – but as the years go by he will meet others on similar paths and his true purpose will be revealed to him. However, what he is going through now is nothing in comparison to the pain and torment he was suffering. He has gained an inner strength and peace and an understanding that will hopefully enable him to reach his potential and make a difference during his time on this planet.

Tom is another male client who had to contend with a strong father who struggled to associate feminine, creative qualities with his image of masculinity. For Tom to be a writer, and to learn to feel comfortable in that career, has entailed a lot of soul searching and hard work. I'm looking forward to seeing his success as he taps into his true feminine creativity and leaves behind his past conditioning. Here, Tom tells his own story.

Tom's story

'I suppose I'd felt for some time that looking more closely at what I ate could be helpful in my healing process, but it was seeing the dramatic improvement in my partner's health that provided the final impetus.

I had been involved in personal development and had used alternative therapies for a number of years but I was still regularly suffering from debilitating and extremely painful headaches.

I teach scriptwriting and have had a great deal of success in "turning on" lots of students to the joys of creative writing. However, despite consistent confirmation of my own ability as a writer, I have suffered a good deal of ambivalence, as well as a lack of confidence, about my own work.

At the end of our first session, Barbara asked me how I felt with what she had suggested. I can still remember the hubris with which I shrugged the question off. This was no big deal to an evolved guy like me who already ate fairly healthily. Knowing the power of dramatic irony only too well, part of me looks back with amusement at that cock-sure attitude. I found myself having sudden fits of rage, cursing vegetables and hurling the sieve across the kitchen as I drained yet another load of brown rice. I was also astonished at how these outbursts seem to come from nowhere.

Sticking with the discipline of the nutritional programme was sometimes far from easy and it is to Barbara's credit that she knew just when and how to offer support. She sensitively worked her holistic magic, addressing mind, body and spirit. As the detoxification continued, I found greater equilibrium: my health started to improve and my headaches lessened. In particular my energy levels and my moods evened out. I found a more naturally-rooted zest for living coming up. I could make changes in circumstances faster and more easily, and there was a pronounced improvement in knowing what I wanted and being able to assert those wishes, as well as being able to break patterns of over-adaptation to others.

There have been major changes in my life: my relationship broke up; a much postponed plan to redecorate my house has been acted upon; my teaching work has changed direction; I have started training as a drama therapist; I have started offering personal development/creativity workshops; and I have now (18 months on) started a new relationship that feels much easier than previous liaisons.

Working with Barbara has been a significant experience in my life. It has helped me to discover a more solid sense of self-worth, an inner knowing of what I need, along with a deeper impulse to really care for myself – and I'm now starting to feel a new dawn looming on the creative writing front.'

Hopefully by reading my story, and those of some of my clients, you will have gained some insight into the extent to which dietary measures can improve not only our physical health, but also our mental and emotional state. If you are having health problems why not try a change of diet? If you feel lost and don't know what direction to take in life, a change of diet might help you find yourself. If you are having problems with a relationship or work colleagues then what have you to lose by changing your diet? Good luck and may you find your path, your potential and your health.

Some guidance on recipes and ingredients

Serving size: I decided to make most of the recipes in this book feed two people, rather than four as in my previous books. This makes it easier for those of you who are cooking for one, as I know is often the case. The recipes are easy to halve for one, or double if you are cooking for four or want extra for the next day or the freezer. The soups still feed four as they all freeze so easily. I have tried to suggest lots of alternatives where possible in recipes, so that readers can work around likes and dislikes as well as allergies and intolerances.

Tablespoons and teaspoons: The spoons I have used when creating these recipes are measuring spoons.

Milk: Where recipes contain milk I have used soya milk, but others could be substituted. The choice is now wide and includes milk made from ingredients such as oats, rice, quinoa and almonds. However, while some milks are naturally sweet, others have sweeteners such as apple juice added and these would be less acceptable in savoury recipes. I've not been able to test all the milks available in all the recipes so take care as some may separate on heating.

Yogurt: Where recipes contain yogurt I have used soya yogurt, but this can often be replaced with goat or sheep's yogurt or even coconut milk.

Soya Dream: I have suggested this as an alternative to cream for serving with desserts. It's made from soya beans but does have fructose and glucose syrup added. It is readily available in supermarkets and health food shops.

Tomatoes: If necessary, tinned tomatoes can be replaced with carrot juice or stock, or even tinned lentils in some vegetarian dishes. Tomato purée can be omitted and other vegetables used instead of fresh tomatoes.

Lemon juice and lemon rind: I have used lemon juice and lemon rind to flavour some recipes but they could be omitted without too much detriment to the flavour. Vinegar can be used in salad dressings, if you do not have a problem with fermented foods, or another fruit juice, such as orange or pineapple, added. I like to freeze both lemon juice and lemon rind so that they are always to hand. I place the grated rind in containers and provided you don't press it down, it's easy to extract a teaspoon when needed. I freeze the juice in ice cube trays then decant into a storage container once frozen.

Pickled lemons: Whole lemons are preserved in brine and provide a wonderful Moroccan flavouring to dishes. Omit if you cannot tolerate citrus. For suppliers see the list at the back of this book.

Fruit juices: These can be substituted with other juices – try pineapple juice instead of orange juice and apple juice instead of grape.

Tamari sauce: This is a wheat-free alternative to soya sauce. It imparts a wonderful savoury flavour to recipes, but it is fermented, so avoid if you have Candida problems. It is useful for adding to dishes you feel are lacking in flavour, and is readily available in health food shops and some supermarkets.

Fish sauce: This adds a wonderful flavour to any savoury dishes and doesn't really smell or taste fishy. It is made from anchovies, salt and 2 per cent sugar. It is fermented, so avoid it if you have Candida problems. Suppliers are listed at the back of the book, though it is now available in most supermarkets.

Horseradish sauce: A salt-pickled version, containing no dairy produce, is available. See the list of suppliers. This is not fermented, though a little lactic acid may be produced when it is processed. I also found a hot horse-radish in my supermarket that was similar.

Mustard powder: This is available free from wheat in some supermarkets. See also the list of suppliers at the back of this book.

Tamarind: The type of thick dark paste of pure tamarind that I use imparts a tangy lemon flavour to dishes. Again, see the list of suppliers.

Lemon grass: This woody stem is available fresh in oriental grocers and some supermarkets, and also freeze-dried in spice jars. The outer tougher leaves are removed and the centre used to impart a spicy lemon flavour. I buy and freeze it when it is available, so that I always have some to hand.

Chillies: Fresh chillies are readily available in supermarkets. If, like me, you don't like too much heat then avoid the really small chillies as the smaller they are the hotter they tend to be. I buy and freeze chillies, cut in half and deseeded.

Ginger: Although readily available in supermarkets, I like to peel fresh ginger and place in a plastic bag in the freezer. It can then be grated from frozen. This saves you trying to extract ginger from a mouldy, dried-up root that has lain too long in the fridge. If you cannot tolerate ginger, omit this from recipes.

Carob chocolate: The supplier of the one I've used is listed at the back of the book. It contains carob powder, non-hydrogenated vegetable fat, soya powder and lecithin. It comes in plain, orange or peppermint flavours and is quite delicious.

Molasses: This is used as an optional sweetener in some cake and pudding recipes. It contains the goodness left over from sugar processing and is a good source of vitamins and minerals. However, it does contain some sugar residue so avoid it if you have Candida problems. It is readily available in health food shops.

Gluten-free flour: The one I used in these recipes is Doves Farm gluten-free flour, which contains rice flour, potato flour, tapioca flour, maize flour and sarassin flour. It is available in some supermarkets and health food shops, or see the list of suppliers at the back of this book.

Carob flour: This is a caffeine-free alternative to cocoa powder. It is available in some health food shops, or see the list of suppliers at the back of this book.

Herbs: I find herbs so useful for adding flavour to recipes. A limited choice of fresh herbs is now available in supermarkets but I also like to keep a wide selection of dried. I often freeze herbs from the garden for winter use. If you pack the herbs loosely in containers, they will crumble easily once frozen so you don't even need to bother chopping them. Some supermarkets sell frozen herbs too, and these are the best substitute for fresh. If you wish to substitute fresh or frozen herbs for dried then 1 tablespoon of fresh or frozen equates to 1 teaspoon of dried. In some recipes I have stated if measurements are meant to be level or rounded spoons – if this is not stated then use a slightly rounded spoon.

Stocking up: The art of making 'cooking without' easy is to be organized, with plenty of ingredients in your cupboards and freezer. I suggest that you go through this book before you start cooking and stock up on any of the dry, tinned or frozen ingredients that you need. It's so off-putting to look through a recipe book and not have the necessary ingredients to make what you want.

Food processor: I have used a food processor in many recipes, particularly for making cakes and puddings. It is my favourite piece of labour-saving equipment. If you don't have one, often a liquidizer or blender will suffice. I haven't listed alternative ways to produce these recipes as I have in my previous books because I wanted to keep recipes as short and simple as possible, but with a little ingenuity you shouldn't find it too difficult.

Oven temperatures: The ones listed are for normal ovens. If you have a fan-assisted oven you will need to lower temperatures by approximately 20°C, 50°F or two gas numbers.

Sweating: This is mentioned at the beginning of many recipes and means cooking slowly at a medium temperature until the vegetables soften. Cooking in oil at higher temperatures is best avoided as it produces toxic substances.

Starters

Griddled Courgettes with Chilli and Garlic Dressing

Serves 2

The griddle pan gives the courgettes lovely brown stripes, which enhances their appearance. However, you could use a frying pan and forgo the stripes. A variety of dressings could be served with the griddled courgettes – try some of those from the salad section.

340g/12oz courgettes	DRESSING:
1 tbsp olive oil	2 tbsp olive oil
	½ red chilli
	1 garlic clove
	1 tbsp lemon juice
	salt and pepper

1 Top and tail the courgettes and slice lengthways into ½cm/¼in strips.
2 Heat a griddle pan and brush the surface with olive oil. Griddle the cour-gette slices for approximately 2 minutes on each side or until just tender. You may have to cook them in two batches, so keep the first ones warm.
3 To make the dressing, deseed and finely dice the red chilli and press the garlic clove. Heat the 2 tablespoons of olive oil in a pan, add the chilli and garlic and cook until soft.
4 Whisk in the lemon juice and season to taste with salt and pepper.
5 Arrange the courgettes attractively on two serving plates and drizzle the dressing over them. Serve at once.

Garlic Courgettes and Mushrooms

Serves 2

This very quick and easy starter also makes a good lunchtime snack if served with salad and, if acceptable, some crusty bread to mop up the juices.

340g/12oz small courgettes	¼ tsp dried thyme or ½ tsp fresh
170g/6oz mushrooms	¼ tsp dried rosemary or ½ tsp fresh
2 spring onions	salt and pepper
1 garlic clove	1 tsp chopped fresh parsley
1 tbsp olive oil	

1 Slice the courgettes and cut the mushrooms into halves or quarters depending on their size.
2 Cut the spring onions into 1cm/½in lengths and press the garlic clove.
3 Heat the oil in a pan and sweat the courgettes, spring onions and garlic until partly cooked. Add the mushrooms, thyme and rosemary and continue to cook until the vegetables are just softened.
4 Season to taste with salt and pepper and serve in individual dishes, garnished with parsley.

Garlic Mushrooms

Follow the above recipe using 455g/1lb mushrooms and miss out the courgettes. If you want garlic mushrooms in a creamy sauce, add 140g/5oz soya yogurt when the mushrooms are just cooked. Heat through and serve.

Purple Sprouting Broccoli with Hollandaise Sauce

Serves 2

Purple sprouting broccoli is available early in the year for a few months. The heads are much smaller than summer broccoli and come with lots of green leaves. It's worth looking out for as it is scrumptious – even without a sauce. If it isn't available, you could break a large head of broccoli into florets. Substitute fresh asparagus or green beans for the broccoli when this is not in season for an equally delicious and simple starter. Make up the sauce ahead of time if you wish, as it is fine served cold with the warm vegetables.

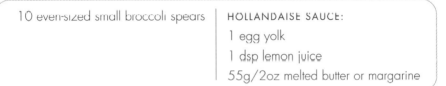

10 even-sized small broccoli spears

HOLLANDAISE SAUCE:

1 egg yolk

1 dsp lemon juice

55g/2oz melted butter or margarine

1   To make the sauce, whisk together the egg yolk and lemon juice and add the melted butter or margarine slowly while continuing to whisk. You can use a processor or blender. Place in a serving jug or dish.
2   Steam the broccoli spears for a few minutes until just tender.
3   Place on warm serving plates and hand round the sauce to accompany.

Antipasto Platter

The ingredients listed below can all be used to make up a platter of your choice. Choose about six from the list. Arrange your selection attractively on two plates and serve. For a light lunch, serve with a green salad and bread or rice cakes.

artichoke hearts	cooked green beans
sunblush or sun-dried tomatoes	roasted peppers
green or black olives	cherry tomatoes
anchovies	celery
tinned or bottled sardines	radish
smoked salmon	avocado
prawns	watercress
crab	tinned sweetcorn
tuna fish	cheese such as buffalo mozzarella or
hard-boiled eggs	feta (if acceptable)
pâté	

Avocado Pear with Ginger Dressing
Serves 2

For a sophisticated start to a meal try this salad of pear and avocado. Its taste and looks belie the simple ingredients and ease of preparation.

DRESSING:	salt and pepper
½ tsp grated orange rind	
60ml/2fl oz fresh orange juice	1 ripe avocado
1 level tsp mustard powder	1 ripe pear
1 level tsp honey (optional)	mixed lettuce leaves (to include rocket)
2 tbsp olive oil	walnuts to garnish
¼ tsp ground ginger or ½ tsp grated fresh ginger	

1 Whisk together the dressing ingredients.
2 Peel and stone the avocado, and peel and core the pear. Cut each into eight segments. Divide the lettuce leaves between two plates and place the pear slices on top, alternating the two types.
3 Pour over the dressing and garnish with a few chopped walnuts. Serve immediately.

Guacamole Dip with Tortilla Chips
Serves 2

This is quite a mild version of guacamole so add more chillies if you want more heat. It is a refreshing dip that is also good served with fresh vegetable crudités or with oatcakes, rice cakes or Melba toast, if you cannot eat corn.

2 ripe avocados	1 tbsp chopped fresh coriander
1 tbsp lemon juice	salt and pepper
2 large ripe tomatoes	coriander leaves to garnish
½ red chilli or a few drops of Tabasco sauce	tortilla chips to serve

1 Peel and stone the avocados and place the flesh in a bowl. Add the lemon juice and roughly mash with a fork.
2 Skin and finely chop the tomatoes (place in boiling water for a few seconds to loosen the skins). Finely dice the chilli if using. Add the tomato and chilli or Tabasco sauce to the avocado and mix well.
3 Mix in the chopped coriander and season to taste with salt and pepper.
4 Garnish the guacamole with fresh coriander and serve with tortilla chips.

Smoked Trout
with Horseradish Dressing

Serves 2

When buying smoked fish try to find a variety that has been naturally smoked. If you wish, you can substitute mackerel or sardines in this recipe – as well as smoked mackerel and fresh sardines try tinned and bottled varieties. The supermarkets are producing some really delicious options now. See the list of suppliers for a source of horseradish, though I found an acceptable bottled hot horseradish in my local supermarket.

mixed salad leaves	salt and pepper
2 small smoked trout fillets	lemon wedges and paprika to garnish
6 tbsp soya (or other) yogurt	
2 tbsp grated horseradish, fresh or bottled	

1 Lay the salad leaves on two plates and place the trout fillets on top.
2 Mix together the yogurt and horseradish and season to taste with salt and pepper. Drizzle the dressing over the fish and salad.
3 Garnish with lemon wedges and a sprinkle of paprika before serving.

Savoury Fruit Salad

Serves 2

I first created this salad when friends arrived unexpectedly one afternoon. We sat on the patio in the summer sunshine, relishing every mouthful. Lots of other fruit and vegetables can be substituted in this recipe. Try baby broad beans and fresh peas or melon and raspberries. In winter, try pineapple, sharon fruit, mango and fresh dates.

1 stick celery	6 strawberries
10cm/4in piece cucumber	2 tbsp French Dressing (see page 72)
½ peach	1dsp chopped fresh mint
½ pear	mint leaves to garnish
½ apple	

1 Cut the vegetables and fruit into bite-sized pieces and mix them in a bowl.
2 Toss in the French dressing and chopped mint. Allow to stand for 15 minutes for the flavours to mingle.
3 Serve in individual glasses decorated with the mint leaves.

Melon and Strawberries
with Strawberry Coulis

Serves 2

Add a little honey to the coulis if it is not sweet enough, provided that honey is acceptable.

¼ melon – gala, honeydew etc.	1 tsp lemon juice
225g/8oz strawberries	

1 Peel and deseed the melon and cut into 6 slices. Hull and wash the strawberries. Cut the strawberries into pieces if large.
2 Place the melon slices on two serving plates with half of the strawberries.
3 Process the remaining strawberries with the lemon juice to produce a smooth coulis.
4 Pour the coulis around the fruit on the plates and serve.

Fresh Pineapple with Raspberry Coulis

Follow the above recipe using wedges of pineapple instead of melon, and raspberries instead of strawberries. Omit the lemon juice and sieve the processed raspberries to remove the seeds.

Fresh Figs with Blackberry Coulis

Serve the figs halved and make the blackberry coulis in the same way as the raspberry.

Fresh Mango with Blueberry Coulis

Serve slices of fresh mango with a blueberry coulis. Make the coulis as described above, using blueberries and lemon juice, but do not sieve the coulis to remove the blueberry skins as they are full of goodness.

Spinach and Cashew Nut Pâté

Serves 4

I love pâtés. I find them so easy to make and so useful to have in the fridge. They're super with salad for lunch or spread on oatcakes or rice cakes to serve with soup. They can be used for afternoon snacks or suppers and make a delightful filling for baked potatoes or sandwiches. They also freeze well.

170g/6oz baby spinach leaves	½ tsp grated nutmeg
115g/4oz cashews	salt and pepper

1 Wash the spinach and steam or cook in the water left on the leaves from washing – do not over-cook the spinach or it will lose its bright green colour. Allow the spinach to cool a little and then squeeze to remove any excess moisture.

2 Process the cashews nuts until finely ground and then add the spinach and nutmeg. Process again, until smooth.

3 Season to taste with salt and pepper and serve with rice cakes or oatcakes and a salad garnish.

Butterbean and Thyme Pâté

Serves 4

If you use tinned butterbeans and dried thyme this pâté takes minutes to make. It is based on a Greek recipe. The butterbeans absorb the olive oil in the same way that egg yolks do when making mayonnaise and the result is a light and tasty pâté that isn't at all oily.

1 garlic clove	1 level tsp grated lemon rind
225g/8oz cooked butterbeans	60ml/2fl oz olive oil
1 tbsp fresh thyme or 1 tsp dried thyme	Salt and pepper
1 tbsp lemon juice	

1 Press the garlic clove and process with the beans, thyme, lemon juice and lemon rind.
2 With the processor switched on, slowly drizzle the oil in through the funnel and continue to process until well combined.
3 Season to taste with salt and pepper and serve with rice cakes or oatcakes and a salad garnish.

Spiced Carrot Dip
with Vegetable Crudités

Serves 4

This delicious dip has a sweet and spicy flavour. It can also be used as a pâté and freezes well.

455g/1lb carrots (weighed after peeling)	2fl oz olive oil
½ tsp ground cumin	salt and pepper
½ tsp paprika	
¼ tsp ground ginger or 1 tsp grated fresh ginger	CRUDITÉS: sticks of celery and cucumber, whole
1 tbsp lemon juice	cherry tomatoes, slices of pepper and
½ tsp lemon rind	courgettes, tortilla chips, baby rice
1 tbsp chopped fresh coriander	cakes etc.

1 Cut the carrots into slices then simmer until cooked. Sieve to remove the cooking liquid and allow them to cool.
2 Process the carrots with the cumin, paprika, ginger, lemon juice, lemon rind and the fresh coriander until smooth.
3 With the processor still running, drizzle in the olive oil through the funnel and process to combine.
4 Season to taste with salt and pepper and serve with the crudités.

Sun-dried Tomato and Lentil Pâté
Serves 4

Sun-dried tomatoes are available dried or bottled in olive oil. The dried ones can be a little tough but their flavour is excellent. If using these, place them on top of the lentils halfway through cooking. They will absorb the steam and soften.

1 onion	10 sun-dried tomatoes
2 garlic cloves	2 tbsp tomato purée
1 tbsp olive oil	1 heaped tsp dried basil or 1 tbsp
170g/6oz red split lentils	chopped fresh basil
400ml/14fl oz boiling water	salt and pepper

1 Finely dice the onion and press the garlic cloves. Sweat these in the olive oil until the onion begins to soften and brown.
2 Wash the lentils and add to the pan along with the boiling water. Cover and simmer over a low heat until the mixture becomes a thick purée and the water has been absorbed. This will take approximately 30–40 minutes.
3 Process the lentil and onion mixture with the sun-dried tomatoes, tomato purée and basil until smooth.
4 Season to taste with salt and pepper and serve with rice cakes or oatcakes and a salad garnish.

Chicken and Walnut Pâté

Serves 4

This is a useful pâté for using up leftover cooked chicken. If you haven't any, then gently sauté a chicken breast in a little olive oil until cooked.

115g/4oz cooked chicken	1 level tsp dried tarragon or 1 tbsp
85g/3oz walnuts	chopped fresh tarragon
4 tbsp soya yogurt	salt and pepper
4 tbsp soya milk	1 tbsp chopped walnuts to garnish

1 Cut the chicken into pieces and process with the walnuts, soya yogurt, soya milk and tarragon until combined but not too smooth.
2 Season to taste with salt and pepper, garnish with chopped walnuts and serve.

Fried Peaches and Pine Nuts
on a Rocket Salad

Serves 2

This recipe features some wonderful combinations of textures and flavours, as well as the contrast of warm peaches on cool salad leaves. It has become one of my favourite starters.

2 ripe medium peaches	1 tbsp fresh basil leaves
1 tsp olive oil	1 tbsp mint leaves
mixed salad leaves (to include rocket)	Olive oil or French Dressing (see page
2 tbsp toasted pine nuts	72)

1 Cut the peaches in half, remove the stones and dry the cut sides on kitchen paper. Fry the peach halves cut side down in the olive oil until heated through and beginning to brown.
2 Place the salad leaves on two plates and place the peaches on top, cut side uppermost.
3 Sprinkle with the pine nuts and torn leaves of basil and mint.
4 Dress with a little good quality olive oil or French Dressing and serve at once.

Grapefruit, Crab and Avocado Starter

Serves 2

Although this recipe is nicer with fresh crab and grapefruit, you can use tinned grapefruit in natural fruit juice and tinned crab meat. As a variation try using cooked prawns instead of the crab or mango instead of the grapefruit.

1 avocado	1 level tsp mustard
1 grapefruit	2 tbsp grapefruit juice (squeeze the
mixed salad leaves (to include	grapefruit membrane or a few segments
watercress)	to produce this)
115g/4oz white crab meat	salt and pepper
2 tbsp olive oil	

1 Peel and stone the avocado and cut into slices.
2 Peel and segment the grapefruit.
3 Divide the salad leaves between two plates and arrange the avocado, grapefruit and crab meat on top.
4 Mix together the olive oil, mustard and grapefruit juice.
5 Season the dressing to taste with salt and pepper and drizzle it over the salad before serving.

Smoked Salmon and Asparagus Salad
Serves 2

When asparagus is not in season, try substituting cooked green beans or avocado. If you wish, you could use a French dressing (see page 72) instead of the olive and herb dressing in this recipe.

1 small bunch asparagus	1 tbsp chopped fresh mixed herbs (i.e.
2 slices smoked salmon	chives, parsley, mint, tarragon, lemon
6 cherry tomatoes	balm, fennel)
mixed salad leaves	4 tbsp olive oil
	Salt and pepper

1   Steam the asparagus until just tender. Allow it to cool then cut the spears into bite-sized pieces.
2   Cut the smoked salmon into pieces and halve the cherry tomatoes.
3   Place the salad leaves on two plates and arrange the asparagus, smoked salmon and tomatoes on top.
4   Mix the chopped herbs with the olive oil and season to taste with salt and pepper. Drizzle the dressing over the salad and serve at once.

Avocado Pear with Prawns

Serves 2

This is a starter that has stood the test of time but sometimes we overlook the obvious when looking for interesting recipes. What could be simpler or more delicious than this to start a meal, or add a salad and serve for a light lunch? If you don't want to use the soya yogurt dressing then use French Dressing instead (see page 72).

DRESSING:	salt and pepper
6 tbsp soya yogurt	
½ tsp mustard	115g/4oz cooked prawns
1 spring onion	1 large avocado

1   Mix the yogurt with the mustard. Dice the spring onion very finely, saving a little of the green part of the onion to garnish, and add to the yogurt mixture.
2   Season the dressing to taste with salt and pepper. Set a few of the prawns aside as a garnish and mix the remainder into the dressing.
3   Peel and stone the avocado and cut into slices. Place the slices onto two serving plates, arranging them in a fan shape.
4   Pile the dressed prawns onto the plates and garnish with the remaining prawns and chopped spring onion.

Pear, Pine Nut and Sun-dried Tomatoes with Ginger Yogurt Dressing

Serves 2

If you intend to use dried sun-dried tomatoes in this recipe, rather than those bottled in olive oil, soak them first in boiling water for approximately 15 minutes so that they plump up and soften. If you don't want to use soya yogurt in the dressing then add the ginger and honey to some olive oil or French dressing.

mixed salad leaves	DRESSING:
2 medium, ripe pears	4 tbsp soya yogurt
4 sun-dried tomatoes	1 tsp grated fresh ginger
2 tbsp toasted pine nuts	1 tsp runny honey (optional)
	salt and pepper

1 Place the salad leaves on two plates.
2 Peel, core and quarter the pears and place on top of the leaves.
3 Cut the sun-dried tomatoes into small pieces and sprinkle over the pears along with the pine nuts, saving a few of each as a garnish.
4 To make the dressing, combine the yogurt with the ginger and honey and season to taste with salt and pepper. Add a little water if necessary to make a runny dressing. Drizzle the dressing over the salad.
5 Garnish with the remaining sun-dried tomatoes and pine nuts and serve.

Soups

Soups are very adaptable when it comes to substituting ingredients so don't be afraid of trying something different – you may just invent a better recipe. I always start soup recipes with an onion, but miss this out if you cannot tolerate onions. Soups don't have to be processed so it doesn't matter if you don't have a processor.

Soups do, however, need good stock. I often make my own from chicken carcasses. If I see organic chickens for sale, I often buy three. I then remove the legs and breasts and freeze these for use at a later date. I roast the carcasses upside down, in a roasting tin, in 570ml/1 pint of water. Once cooked and cooled, I remove any meat from the carcasses and use this for a curry, soup or any other dish requiring cooked chicken. I then boil the carcasses in 2.8 litres/5 pints of water for about an hour, then sieve and cool the stock in the fridge overnight. Any fat that comes to the surface can be easily removed as the stock sets to a jelly – for this I use a few thicknesses of kitchen paper pressed onto the surface. The fat soaks into or sticks to it and is lifted away when you remove the paper. The stock can then be frozen in containers for future use. It is a bit of a chore but worth it for the excellent stock it provides.

Stocks, including chicken and vegetable, can be bought fresh from the chiller cabinets in the supermarket but they are quite expensive. Miso, preferably light miso, makes good stock and tamari sauce is a useful addition for soups that are lacking in flavour. However, both these are fermented foods and will not be suitable for Candida sufferers. Failing any of the above I resort to yeast-free stock cubes, but as I'm not too happy with the manufacturing process which these go through, I try to limit their use. If you do use them, be careful not to add much salt, as they are usually quite salty.

I have used soya milk in these recipes but other milks could be substituted. Do not use any that contain added sweeteners or they will spoil the taste of the soup. Soya milk can separate a little if over-cooked so try to avoid this once the milk has been added to the soup.

Sweating the vegetables at the beginning of most recipes can be missed out if time is short or you prefer not to do this. The flavour of the soup will suffer a little but it will still be quite acceptable.

Spinach, Potato and Celery Soup
Serves 4

This soup has a delicate colour, a rich creamy texture and a subtle flavour.

1 large onion	225g/8oz spinach
170g/6oz celery	1 tbsp chopped fresh tarragon or 1 tsp
1 tbsp olive oil	dried tarragon
285g/10oz potatoes	½ tsp grated nutmeg
1.1 litres/2 pints stock (vegetable or	285ml/½ pint soya milk
chicken)	salt and pepper

1 Finely dice the onion and celery and sweat these in the olive oil until they begin to soften.
2 Grate the potatoes and add to the pan along with the stock. Bring to the boil and simmer until the onions, celery and potatoes are cooked.
3 Add the spinach, tarragon and nutmeg, bring to the boil again and simmer for 5 minutes.
4 Process the soup until smooth.
5 Add the soya milk, salt and pepper to taste and heat through before serving. Do not continue to cook the soup or the spinach will lose its bright green colour and the soya milk may start to separate.

Courgette, Rosemary and Garlic Soup
Serves 4

Courgettes can produce a rather bland soup, but not in this case. This soup really is delightful, with a wonderful combination of flavours. I often make it at the end of summer when we have a glut of courgettes in the garden. It freezes well and is a reminder of summer days.

2 onions	1.4 litres/2½ pints stock (vegetable or
2 garlic cloves	chicken)
1 tbsp olive oil	2 rounded tsp fresh chopped rosemary
4 courgettes	or 1 tsp dried rosemary
1 medium potato	2 tbsp chopped fresh parsley
	salt and pepper

1 Finely dice the onions and press the garlic cloves.
2 Sweat these in the olive oil until they begin to soften and brown.
3 Grate the courgettes and potato and add to the pan, along with the stock and rosemary. Bring to the boil and simmer for 10 minutes then process the soup until smooth.
4 Add the parsley and salt and pepper to taste. Bring to the boil and serve.

Cauliflower and Ginger Soup
Serves 4

Rich and satisfying, this tasty and nutritious soup is warming on a chilly winter's day.

1 medium head of cauliflower	1.4 litres/2½ pints stock (vegetable or chicken)
1 large onion	
4cm/1½in piece ginger	salt and pepper
1 tbsp olive oil	parsley to garnish

1　Break the cauliflower into small florets, dice the onion and grate the ginger.
2　Sweat these in the olive oil until they begin to soften.
3　Add the stock, bring to the boil and simmer until the cauliflower is just cooked.
4　Process the soup, add salt and pepper to taste and warm through before serving. Garnish with chopped parsley.

Chicken and Vegetable Soup
with Butterbeans and Barley
Serves 4

This is a real down-to-earth soup that provides a substantial meal in itself. I often make it when I have a chicken carcass to use up. I sometimes cook the barley with the chicken while making the stock. At other times I cook a large batch of barley (this takes about 40 minutes in boiling water) and then freeze it in small quantities for use in soups and casseroles. Other beans can be substituted for the butterbeans.

1 onion	115g/4oz cooked barley
1 medium carrot	400g tin butterbeans
¼ celeriac or 1 parsnip	1.4 litres/2½ pints chicken stock
2 sticks celery	2 tbsp chopped fresh parsley
¼ small cabbage or 2 courgettes	salt and pepper
115g/4oz cooked chicken	

1 Dice the vegetables and place in the pan with the chicken, barley, butter-beans and stock.
2 Bring to the boil and simmer until all the vegetables are cooked. This will take approximately 20 minutes.
3 Add the parsley, salt and pepper to taste and serve.

Pumpkin and Prawn Creole

Serves 4

This soup is full of robust flavours. I love to make it in the autumn, when pumpkins first come into the shops, as it seems to help compensate for the passing of summer. Butternut squash or sweet potatoes can be substituted for the pumpkin.

1 large onion	½ level tsp dried thyme
2 medium carrots	2 tbsp tomato purée (optional)
1 leek	1.4 litres/2½ pints stock (vegetable or
1 tbsp olive oil	chicken)
565g/1¼lb pumpkin flesh	140g/5oz frozen cooked prawns
1 rounded tsp paprika	salt and pepper
1 rounded tsp dried oregano	toasted sesame seeds to garnish

1   Dice the onion and carrots and slice the leek. Sweat the vegetables in the olive oil until they begin to soften.
2   Cube the pumpkin flesh. You do not need to peel the pumpkin unless the skin is blemished or old and starting to go tough.
3   Add the pumpkin to the pan and continue to sweat the vegetables, stirring regularly, until the pumpkin flesh starts to soften.
4   Add the paprika, oregano, thyme and tomato purée and mix in.
5   Add the stock and bring to the boil. Simmer until the vegetables are soft.
6   Process the soup until smooth.
7   Add the prawns and salt and pepper to taste. Heat through and serve garnished with the sesame seeds.

Chicken Noodle Soup

Serves 4

This is a nutritious and delicious soup. It is another good recipe to make with the remains of a chicken, although it is also fine made with chicken breast meat.

1 large onion	1 bay leaf
1 garlic clove	326g tin sweetcorn in water
1 tbsp olive oil	1 tbsp chopped fresh parsley
140g/5oz chicken	1 tbsp tamari sauce (optional)
1.4 litres/2½ pints chicken stock	salt and pepper
85g/3oz fine rice noodles	

1 Dice the onion and press the garlic clove.
2 Sweat these in the olive oil until they begin to soften.
3 Dice the chicken and add to the pan. If using fresh chicken, cook until coloured.
4 Add the stock, noodles and bay leaf and bring to the boil. Simmer until the noodles and chicken are tender, approximately 10 minutes.
5 Add the sweetcorn, parsley, tamari sauce and salt and pepper to taste.
6 Remove the bay leaf, heat through and serve.

Leek, Mint and Almond Soup
Serves 4

The unusual combination of flavours in this recipe works well to produce a hearty soup. It is thickened by the addition of ground almonds but these could be omitted for a less substantial version of this soup.

1 medium onion	1.1 litres/2 pints stock (vegetable or
680g/1½lb leeks	chicken)
1 tbsp olive oil	285ml/½ pint soya milk
handful fresh mint leaves or 1 tbsp	55g/2oz ground almonds
chopped frozen mint	salt and pepper
1 tbsp fresh tarragon or 1 tsp dried	

1 Dice the onion and slice the leeks.
2 Sweat these in the olive oil until they begin to soften and brown.
3 Add the mint, tarragon and stock. Bring to the boil and simmer until the vegetables are cooked – approximately 5 minutes.
4 Process the soup until smooth.
5 Add the soya milk and ground almonds and heat through. Season the soup to taste with salt and pepper and serve. Do not continue to cook the soup or the soya milk may start to separate.

Parsnip, Ginger and Orange Soup

Serves 4

Nearly all root vegetables make excellent soup, as they purée well and have a wonderful flavour. The warmth that the ginger imparts makes this an excellent soup for chilly winter days.

1 large onion	juice of 2 oranges (approx.
1 garlic clove	140ml/5fl oz)
2 tbsp olive oil	1.4 litres/2½ pints vegetable or
455g/1lb parsnips	chicken stock
225g/½lb carrots	salt and pepper
1½in piece ginger	2 tbsp chopped fresh parsley to
1 tsp grated orange rind	garnish

1 Dice the onion and press the garlic clove then sweat these in the olive oil until the onion begins to soften.
2 Peel and grate the parsnips, carrots and ginger and add them to the pan. Continue to sweat the vegetables until the parsnips and carrots begin to soften.
3 Add the orange rind and juice and the stock. Bring to the boil and simmer for another 10 minutes or until all the ingredients are cooked.
4 Process the soup.
5 Season to taste with salt and pepper, heat through and serve garnished with parsley.

Smoked Haddock Chowder
Serves 4

This recipe produces a thick 'meal-in-itself' soup that is full of delicious flavours. Use naturally smoked haddock, which is available in most fish-mongers.

1 onion	1 bay leaf
2 medium leeks	1 level tsp dried thyme or 1 tbsp fresh
4 sticks celery	455g/1lb smoked haddock
2 large potatoes	1 rounded tbsp corn or rice flour
1 garlic clove	285ml/½ pint soya milk
1 tbsp olive oil	2 tbsp chopped parsley
1.1 litres/2 pints stock (vegetable or fish)	salt and pepper

1 Dice the onion, slice the leeks and celery, and cut the potatoes into chunks. Press the garlic clove. Sweat these in the olive oil until they begin to soften.

2 Add the stock, bay leaf and thyme, bring to the boil and simmer until the vegetables are just cooked.

3 Cut the smoked haddock into small pieces and add to the soup. Bring to the boil and simmer for 5 minutes.

4 Mix the flour with the soya milk and add to the pan, along with the parsley. Bring to the boil, stirring constantly, and simmer for 1 minute. Do not over-cook the soup at this stage or the soya milk may separate a little.

5 Season the soup to taste with salt and pepper, remove the bay leaf and serve.

Cream of Celery Soup
Serves 4

This is an old favourite that I've updated. Celery produces wonderful soup with an excellent flavour and appearance.

1 onion	¼ tsp dried thyme or ½ tsp fresh
1 medium head of celery	2 dsp corn or rice flour
1 tbsp olive oil	285ml/½ pint soya milk
1.1 litres/2 pints stock (vegetable or chicken)	1 tbsp chopped fresh parsley
1 bay leaf	salt and pepper
1 tsp celery seeds	chopped parsley to garnish

1 Dice the onion and finely slice the celery.
2 Sweat the onion and celery in the olive oil until they begin to soften and brown.
3 Add the stock, bay leaf, celery seeds and thyme. Bring to the boil and simmer until the vegetables are cooked.
4 Process the soup mixture until fairly smooth. I like to find a few pieces of celery left whole, so don't over-process the soup unless you want it completely smooth.
5 Mix the flour with the milk and add to the soup along with the parsley. Bring to the boil, stirring constantly, and simmer for 1 minute. Do not continue to cook or the soya milk may start to separate.
6 Season to taste with salt and pepper, remove the bay leaf and serve garnished with the remaining chopped parsley.

Fish Soup

Serves 4

This delicious and nutritious soup is an ideal way to serve fish to those who are nervous of bones. You can make sure they are all removed as you flake or cut up the fish.

1 large onion	1 tsp dried dill or 1 tbsp fresh
2 sticks celery	½ tsp dried tarragon or 1 dsp fresh
1 large carrot	1 tsp fennel seeds
1 large leek	225g/8oz white fish e.g. cod
1 garlic clove	85g/3oz frozen prawns
1 tbsp olive oil	1 tbsp fish sauce (optional)
1.1 litres/2 pints fish or vegetable stock	1 tbsp corn or rice flour
	285ml/½ pint soya milk
½ tsp celery seeds	salt and pepper

1   Dice the onion, celery and carrot, slice the leek and press the garlic clove.
2   Sweat the vegetables and garlic in the olive oil until they begin to soften.
3   Add the stock, celery seeds, dill, tarragon and fennel seeds. Bring to the boil and simmer until the vegetables are just cooked.
4   Cut or flake the fish into bite sized pieces and add to the pan along with the prawns and fish sauce. Bring to the boil and simmer for 2 minutes or until the fish is cooked.
5   Mix the flour with the milk and add to the pan. Bring the soup to the boil again, stirring constantly. Simmer for 1 minute but do not continue to cook or the soya milk may separate a little and the fish will become tough.
6   Season to taste if necessary (you won't need salt if using fish sauce) and serve.

Tomato, Lentil and Mint Soup

Serves 4

This is a really quick and easy soup to make, using ingredients that are usually at hand. Even if you don't sweat the onions, you will still obtain a very acceptable soup.

2 large onions	850ml/1½ pints stock (vegetable or
1 tbsp olive oil	chicken)
115g/4oz red split lentils	2 dsp chopped fresh or frozen mint
2 x 425g tins chopped tomatoes	salt and pepper

1   Dice the onions and sweat them slowly in the olive oil until they begin to soften and brown.
2   Wash the lentils and add to the pan along with the tomatoes and stock. Bring to the boil and simmer until the lentils are soft. This will take approximately 20 minutes.
3   Process the soup until smooth.
4   Add the mint and simmer for 2 minutes. Season the soup to taste with salt and pepper and serve.

Butterbean, Spinach and Lemon Soup
Serves 4

A combination of butterbeans, potatoes and spinach is puréed to produce this exceedingly tasty soup.

2 onions	225g/8oz spinach
1 tbsp olive oil	2 dsp lemon juice
1 medium potato	2 tsp grated lemon rind
1.4 litres/2½ pints stock (vegetable or chicken)	½ tsp ground nutmeg
	salt and pepper
400g tin butterbeans	4 tbsp soya yogurt to garnish

1 Dice the onions and sweat them in the olive oil until they begin to soften.
2 Dice the potato and add to the pan along with the stock and drained butterbeans. Bring to the boil and simmer until the onions and potato are soft.
3 Add the spinach, lemon juice, lemon rind and nutmeg and simmer for a further 5 minutes. Do not over cook or the spinach will lose its bright green colour.
4 Process the soup until smooth. Season to taste with salt and pepper and serve with a tablespoon of soya yogurt swirled into each bowl.

Beetroot Soup with Mint and Coconut

Serves 4

Over the years I have often tried to make a good beetroot soup but I've never been impressed. This one, however, is something special and it's going to become one of my favourites.

1 large onion	55g/2oz creamed coconut
1 tbsp olive oil	2 dsp lemon juice
2 medium carrots	2 tbsp chopped fresh parsley
565g/1¼lb raw beetroot	2 tbsp chopped fresh mint
1.4 litres/2½ pints stock (vegetable	salt and pepper
or chicken)	4–5 tbsp soya yogurt

1 Dice the onion and sweat it in the olive oil until it begins to soften.
2 Peel the carrots and beetroot then grate them and add to the pan along with the stock.
3 Simmer for 15 minutes or until the vegetables are soft.
4 Cut the block of coconut into small pieces and add to the pan with the lemon juice. Allow the coconut to dissolve and then process the soup until smooth.
5 Add the chopped parsley and mint and season to taste with salt and pepper.
6 Heat the soup again and serve with a spoonful of soya yogurt swirled through each bowl.

Cream of Mushroom Soup

Serves 4

I always find mushroom soup irresistible. This one, with the addition of dried porcini mushrooms, has an intense and satisfying flavour.

10g/½oz porcini mushrooms	850ml/1½ pints stock (vegetable or chicken)
285ml/½ pint boiling water	
1 medium onion	2 dsp corn or rice flour
1 garlic clove	1 tsp mustard
1 tbsp olive oil	285ml/½ pint soya milk
125g/4½oz chestnut mushrooms	salt and pepper
125g/4½oz field mushrooms	1 tbsp chopped fresh parsley

1 Soak the porcini mushrooms in the boiling water.
2 Dice the onion and press the garlic clove. Sweat the onion and garlic in the olive oil until they begin to soften and brown.
3 Roughly chop the chestnut and field mushrooms and add them to the pan. Continue to sweat the vegetables until the mushrooms become soft and release their juices.
4 Remove the porcini mushrooms from the soaking liquid and pour the soaking liquid into the soup, taking care to avoid any gritty pieces that may be at the bottom.
5 Finely dice the porcini mushrooms and add to the pan along with the stock. Bring to the boil and simmer until all the vegetables are cooked – approximately 10 minutes. Process the soup until smooth.
6 Mix together the flour, mustard and the soya milk and pour into the soup. Bring to the boil, stirring constantly, and simmer for 1 minute. Do not over-cook at this stage or the soya milk may start to separate.
7 Season to taste with salt and pepper and serve, garnished with fresh parsley.

Leek and Potato Soup

Serves 4

This mouthwatering soup has stood the test of time. It never dates and is still one of my favourites. That's probably because potatoes and leeks go together so well and produce a hearty broth that is filling and warming on winter days.

4 medium leeks	1.1 litres/2 pints vegetable or chicken stock
1 medium onion	
3 medium potatoes	1 bay leaf
1 tbsp olive oil	285ml/½ pint soya milk
	salt and pepper

1 Slice the leeks and onion and dice the potatoes.
2 Sweat the vegetables in the olive oil until they begin to soften.
3 Add the stock and the bay leaf, bring to the boil and simmer for approximately 20 minutes or until the vegetables are cooked.
4 Remove the bay leaf and process half of the soup. Return the processed soup to the pan along with the milk. Bring to the boil but do not continue to cook or the soya milk may start to separate.
5 Add salt and pepper to taste and serve.

Salads

All the salads in this section are main course salads so they can be served in large, individual salad bowls just as they are or, if appetites require it, with a few new potatoes or some crusty bread. If you wish, they can be served as starters, in which case they'll serve four to six rather than two. It's also nice if you are entertaining more than two people to serve a selection of different salads placed in the centre of the table for a help-yourself affair. Most of the salads have their own dressing but I have included a recipe for French dressing, as this can be made in larger quantities and kept in the fridge for when time is short. I also like to ensure I have a bottle of good quality olive oil to use just for dressing salads. Like wine, the flavour of oil varies tremendously, so try a few until you find the one you like best. Salads respond well to substitutions so if there is an ingredient that you don't like or haven't got, then try something else – you might come up with a better recipe. The only rule is to have fun and enjoy combining different textures and flavours.

French Dressing

If you find this dressing a little sharp, try adding the juice of an orange in place of one of the lemons. You could also use cider vinegar or a mixture of cider and balsamic vinegars instead of the lemon juice – if you do not have a problem with yeast-based foods.

grated rind of 1 lemon	2 tsp mixed dried herbs e.g. dill,
juice of 2 lemons	fennel, fennel seeds, celery seeds,
2 rounded tsp mustard	tarragon, parsley, mint or 2 tbsp
1 heaped tsp honey (optional)	chopped fresh herbs e.g. parsley,
good quality olive oil	chives, tarragon, lemon balm, fennel
	salt and pepper

1 Place the lemon rind, lemon juice, mustard and honey in a screw-topped jar and whisk or shake to combine.
2 Add the olive oil until you have added twice as much oil as the other ingredients.
3 Add the herbs, shake well and season to taste with salt and pepper.
4 Store in the fridge ready for use and use within one month.

Tuna Salad Niçoise

Serves 2

It doesn't matter if some of the ingredients in this salad are still slightly warm when you serve it. It is also equally good cold, which means it can be prepared in advance and assembled quickly when you are ready to eat. You can substitute cooked fresh tuna if you prefer.

680g/1½lb new potatoes	2 large tomatoes
340g/12oz French beans	20 black olives
3 eggs	185g tin tuna
salad leaves	olive oil or French Dressing

1 Cook the new potatoes and steam the beans. Cool the beans in cold water to prevent them overcooking and to preserve their bright green colour.
2 Boil the eggs for approximately 8 minutes so that they are hard-boiled but not too solid. Allow the eggs and potatoes to cool while you prepare the rest of the salad.
3 Arrange the salad leaves in two individual salad bowls. Cut the tomatoes into segments and place on the salads. Peel and quarter the eggs, cut the beans in half and cut the potatoes into bite-sized pieces. Arrange these on the salad leaves along with the olives and flakes of tuna fish.
4 Drizzle olive oil or French Dressing over and serve.

Peach, Pasta and Chicken Salad

Serves 2

Pasta is now available made from lots of alternatives to wheat, such as corn and rice. If you do want to use wheat pasta use less – 115g/4oz should be sufficient. If you don't have cooked chicken, use a chicken breast portion and cook this by steaming or gently sautéing. When fresh peaches are not available, try using fresh mango for an equally delightful salad.

170g/6oz gluten-free pasta	2 small courgettes
3 tbsp French dressing	3 spring onions
225g/8oz cooked chicken	handful fresh basil leaves
2 small fresh peaches	salad leaves
½ red pepper	

1 Cook the pasta and drain. Pour over the French dressing while the pasta is still warm to allow it to soak up the flavours as it cools.
2 Dice the chicken, peaches and red pepper. Grate the courgettes coarsely, slice the spring onions and tear the basil leaves into small pieces. Add these to the pasta and gently mix to combine. Allow the mixture to stand for 10 minutes if possible, to allow the flavours to combine.
3 Place the salad leaves in two individual salad bowls, pile the pasta mix on top and serve.

Chicken, Mango and Broad Bean Salad
Serves 2

The sweet and sour combination of fruit and vegetables works to perfection in this salad. For extra flavour, make up another portion of the dressing and marinate the chicken pieces in this for at least an hour before cooking. Use frozen broad beans if fresh are not available and for a variation on this salad use peach instead of mango.

mixed salad leaves (to include some rocket)	DRESSING:
1 small mango	5 tbsp olive or walnut oil
2 spring onions	½ tsp mustard
6 cherry tomatoes	½ tsp honey (optional)
1 avocado	2 tbsp lemon juice
55g/2oz roasted cashews	salt and pepper
12 black olives	
	2 chicken breasts
	1 tbsp olive oil
	2 handfuls broad beans

1   Place the leaves in two individual salad bowls. Cut the mango flesh into large chunks, finely slice the spring onions, halve the tomatoes and cut the avocado into bite-sized pieces. Save a few pieces of mango to garnish and add the rest of the chopped ingredients to the salads, along with the nuts and olives.
2   Whisk the dressing ingredients together.
3   Cut the chicken breasts into bite-sized pieces and sweat in the olive oil until just cooked.
4   While the chicken is cooking, steam the broad beans for 2 minutes or until the skins begin to split. You can leave the broad beans uncooked if you prefer.
5   Pile the warm chicken and beans on top of the salads, drizzle over the dressing, garnish with the remaining mango pieces and serve at once.

Marinated Tofu and Peanut Salad

Serves 2

The contrasts of colours, tastes and textures make this one of my favourite salads – even my husband, who doesn't normally like tofu, thinks that it's wonderful. The tofu is marinated, tossed in flour and then fried, to produce crunchy cubes that are full of flavour. Other salad ingredients that work well in this recipe include sweetcorn, red onion, celery and finely chopped chilli peppers.

250g/9oz plain tofu	salad leaves
	10cm/4in piece cucumber
MARINADE:	2 large tomatoes
1 level tsp mustard	½ yellow pepper
2.5cm/1in piece ginger, grated	2 handfuls beansprouts
1 pressed garlic clove	1 handful roasted salted peanuts
1 tsp honey (optional)	olive oil for dressing
1 tbsp tamari (optional)	2 tbsp gluten-free flour
2 tbsp olive oil	2 tbsp olive oil
salt and pepper	

1 Cube the tofu and press firmly with kitchen paper to remove the excess moisture. Mix the marinade ingredients together and season (you will not need salt if using the tamari sauce). Toss the marinade with the tofu and leave for 2 hours or longer.

2 Place the salad leaves in two individual salad bowls. Cut the cucumber into strips, the tomatoes into wedges and the pepper into dice.

3 Pile the cucumber, tomatoes, pepper, beansprouts and roasted peanuts onto the salad leaves, saving a few peanuts and pieces of pepper to garnish. Dress the salads with olive oil.

4 Remove the tofu from the marinade and toss it in the flour until lightly coated. Sauté the tofu in 2 tablespoons of olive oil over a medium heat, turning regularly, until golden brown.

5 Pile the warm tofu onto the salads, garnish with the peanuts and pepper and serve at once.

Rice Salad
Serves 2

The variations on this salad are endless, as you can use whatever ingredients you have available. I find rice salad useful to take to work instead of sandwiches or for picnics on days out. I often add frozen peas or sweetcorn, which help to keep the salad cool when travelling and are defrosted before you are ready to eat.

400g/14oz cooked rice (200g/7oz uncooked)	cooked chicken
	cheese
good quality olive oil or French dressing	tofu
	peach
	grapes
Choose at least 8 ingredients from the following list:	apple
	orange
avocado	raisins or sultanas
grated courgette	nuts
grated carrot	seeds
celery	peas
radish	sweetcorn
cucumber	broad beans
tomato	tinned beans e.g. kidney
pepper	olives
red onion	sun-dried tomatoes
spring onions	prawns
watercress	crab
cooked French beans	smoked salmon
sprouted seeds	

1 Place the rice in a large bowl. Cut enough of your chosen ingredients into bite-sized pieces to give you an amount similar to the amount of rice. Add them to the bowl.

2 Dress with olive oil or French dressing and gently mix to combine. Serve piled into individual salad bowls.

Tropical Chicken Salad
Serves 2

If desired, the chicken pieces can be marinated in 2 tablespoons of French dressing or an equal mixture of olive oil and lemon juice flavoured with ½ teaspoon of mustard, and salt and pepper. Use tinned pineapple in fruit juice when fresh fruit is not available. To make a vegetarian version of this succulent salad, use the tofu from the Marinated Tofu and Peanut Salad recipe (see page 76).

2 large sticks celery	DRESSING:
mixed salad leaves (to include watercress)	4 tbsp finely chopped pineapple
2 handfuls beansprouts	4 tbsp chopped fresh tarragon
20 chunks fresh pineapple	1 rounded tsp mustard
1 handful walnuts	1 tbsp lemon juice
2 chicken breasts	3 tbsp olive oil
1 tbsp olive oil	salt and pepper

1 Dice the celery and make two salads in individual salad bowls using the celery, salad leaves, beansprouts, pineapple and the walnuts. Save a few pieces of pineapple and walnuts for a garnish.
2 Whisk together the dressing ingredients.
3 Cut the chicken breasts into bite-sized pieces and sweat these in the olive oil until they begin to brown and are just cooked.
4 Pile the warm chicken on top of the salads, drizzle the dressing over and garnish with the remaining pineapple and walnuts. Serve at once.

Chicken and New Potato Salad
with Anchovy and Olive Tapenade

Serves 2

Fresh tuna steaks are a good substitute for the chicken in this recipe. Leave the steaks whole and cook until the outsides are browning but the insides are still slightly pink.

TAPENADE:	mixed salad leaves (to include rocket)
50g tin anchovy fillets	¼ red onion
10 kalamati black olives	2 sticks celery
1 small garlic clove	10 cooked new potatoes
1 tbsp chopped parsley	6 tbsp sweetcorn
5 tbsp olive oil (to include oil from	handful cooked French beans
anchovies)	2 large chicken breasts
	1 garlic clove
	1 tbsp olive oil

1 To make the tapenade, finely chop the anchovies, olives, garlic and parsley by hand and mix together with the olive oil.
2 Place the salad leaves in individual salad bowls. Slice the red onion, dice the celery and cut the potatoes into bite-sized pieces; add to the salad leaves along with the sweetcorn and French beans.
3 Cut the chicken into small pieces and press the garlic clove. Sweat these in the olive oil until the chicken is cooked and beginning to brown.
4 Pile the warm chicken onto the salads and drizzle over the tapenade. Serve immediately.

Mediterranean Chicken Salad with Pesto Dressing

Serves 2

This light and refreshing salad is equally good made with hard-boiled eggs or tuna fish (either fresh or tinned) instead of chicken.

DRESSING:	10 cherry tomatoes
2 handfuls fresh basil leaves	7.5cm/3in piece cucumber
½ tsp mustard	1 large avocado
1 tbsp lemon juice	3 sun-dried tomatoes
5 tbsp olive oil	10 black olives
salt and pepper	2 chicken breasts
	1 garlic clove
mixed salad leaves	1 tbsp olive oil
1 yellow pepper	

1 To make the dressing, very finely chop the basil leaves and mix with the mustard, lemon juice, olive oil and salt and pepper to taste.

2 Place the salad leaves in two individual salad bowls. Dice the pepper, halve the cherry tomatoes and cut the cucumber into sticks, the avocado into chunks and the sun-dried tomatoes into small pieces. Pile these onto the salad leaves along with the olives, saving a few tomatoes and olives to garnish.

3 Cut the chicken into bite-sized pieces and press the garlic clove. Sweat these in the olive oil until the chicken is cooked and beginning to brown.

4 Pile the warm chicken onto the salads and drizzle the dressing over. Garnish with the tomatoes and olives and serve at once.

Kedgeree Salad

Serves 2

This substantial rice salad is a variation on traditional breakfast kedgeree. The many different flavours combine extremely well.

2 eggs	1 tsp grated lemon rind
1 onion	340g/12oz cooked rice (170g/6oz
1 tbsp olive oil	uncooked)
140g/5oz broad beans (fresh or	125g tin mackerel in olive oil
frozen)	2 tbsp chopped fresh coriander
140g/5oz peas (fresh or frozen)	salad leaves
1 level tsp ground cumin	4 tbsp soya or other yogurt (optional)
1 level tsp ground coriander	fresh coriander to garnish
1 tbsp lemon juice	

1   Boil the eggs for 8 minutes and leave to cool.
2   Finely dice the onion and sweat this in the olive oil until it begins to soften. Add the beans and peas and continue to sweat until they are just cooked or defrosted.
3   Add the cumin and coriander and cook for 2 minutes.
4   Remove from the heat and add the lemon juice, lemon rind and cooked rice. Drain the mackerel, cut it into bite-sized pieces and add the fish pieces to the pan, along with the chopped coriander. Mix gently to combine.
5   Place the salad leaves in two individual salad bowls and pile the rice mixture on top. Place two tablespoons of yogurt in the centre of the rice then peel and quarter the hard-boiled eggs and place around the sides. Garnish with fresh coriander and serve.

Roasted Pepper Salad with Salsa Sauce

Serves 2

This is an unusual selection of ingredients but they combine beautifully to produce a mouthwatering salad. Use tinned beans for ease. Peppers skin reasonably easily once cooked but to make the process even easier, place in a bowl while they're still warm and cover the bowl with clingfilm until the peppers are cool. If you cannot tolerate any kind of yogurt, use extra avocado and mash or process it until smooth.

4 mixed peppers	SALSA SAUCE:
1 large red onion	1 avocado
1 tbsp olive oil	7.5cm/3in piece cucumber
salad leaves	½–1 green chilli
225g/8oz cooked rice	1 tbsp lemon juice
(4oz/115g uncooked)	4 heaped tbsp soya or other yogurt
4 tbsp beans e.g. cannellini	2 tbsp chopped coriander
4 tbsp sweetcorn	2 tbsp water
coriander to garnish	salt and pepper

1 Quarter the peppers and remove the seeds and stalks. Peel the onion and cut into 8 segments. Toss the peppers and onions gently in the olive oil to coat and place on a baking tray. Roast, uncovered, at 200°C/400°F/Gas Mark 6 for 20–25 minutes or until the vegetables are just cooked. Leave to cool.

2 Line two individual salad bowls with the salad leaves.

3 Combine the rice, beans and sweetcorn and pile on top of the leaves, leaving the leaves still visible round the sides of the bowls.

4 To make the salsa sauce, finely dice the avocado, cucumber and chilli and mix with the lemon juice, yogurt, chopped coriander and water. Season to taste with salt and pepper.

5 Pile the salsa on top of the rice, leaving a little rice visible around the edges. Peel the skins from the peppers and pile these and the onions on top of the salad. Garnish with coriander and serve.

Tuna, Bean and New Potato Salad
Serves 2

The onion and pepper in this recipe is raw but I have also made this salad with roasted peppers and onions and it was delicious. If the oven is on and I have peppers to spare I will often pop them in to roast so that they are ready for a salad the next day. Double up on the pepper and onion quantities if you decide to roast them, as they do shrink. Flaked fresh tuna could be used in this salad and diced cucumber or celery substituted for any of the salad vegetables. You could also use pasta instead of potatoes.

¼ red onion	115g/4oz sweetcorn
1 red pepper	12 black olives
1 avocado	2 tbsp olive oil or French dressing
285g/10oz cooked new potatoes	185g tin tuna
115g/4oz tinned white beans	salad leaves (to include watercress)
(cannellini, butter etc.)	parsley to garnish

1   Finely slice the red onion, dice the pepper and avocado and cut the new potatoes into bite-sized pieces.
2   Combine these in a bowl with the beans, sweetcorn, olives and the French dressing. Add the tuna last of all and gently mix, without breaking it up too much.
3   Place the salad leaves in two individual salad bowls and pile the tuna mixture on top. Garnish with parsley and serve.

Potato, Chickpea and Tortilla Salad with Satay Sauce

Serves 2

This appetizing and unusual salad is very easy to prepare. Salted peanuts make a good substitute for the tortilla chips if you cannot tolerate corn, and humous can be used as a dressing instead of the satay sauce (water it down a little to make it runny). Other good substitutions include raisins instead of the apple, cucumber instead of the celery, avocado instead of the potatoes and red pepper instead of the chilli.

SATAY SAUCE:	mixed salad leaves
4 tbsp peanut butter	10 medium cooked new potatoes
4 tbsp coconut milk	2 sticks celery
1 pressed garlic clove	½ apple
1 tbsp lemon juice	½ small red onion
1 level tsp honey (optional)	½ red chilli
1 tsp tamari sauce (optional)	½ x 400g tin chickpeas
2 tbsp hot water	1 bunch coriander
salt and pepper	handful tortilla chips

1 To make the sauce, whisk together all the sauce ingredients, adding salt and pepper to taste. Add a little more water if needed until you have a runny dressing.
2 Place the salad leaves in two individual salad bowls.
3 Cut the new potatoes in halves or quarters, dice the celery and apple, finely slice the red onion, and finely dice the chilli.
4 Arrange the vegetables and drained chickpeas in the salad bowls. Add the coriander leaves and the tortilla chips broken into pieces, saving some of each as a garnish.
5 Drizzle the dressing over the salads and serve at once, garnished with the remaining coriander and tortilla chips.

Thai Beef Salad
Serves 2

Enjoy a taste of the East with this colourful and succulent salad. Use fish sauce instead of the tamari and lemon juice instead of lime if desired. See the list of suppliers (page 211) for a source of bottled horseradish or miss this out and use a full tablespoon of tamari or fish sauce.

DRESSING:	
2 tbsp lime juice	½ yellow pepper
2 tbsp olive oil	4 spring onions
1 heaped tsp bottled horseradish	7cm/3in piece cucumber
½ tbsp tamari sauce (optional)	1 carrot
1 tsp honey (optional)	salad leaves
1 tbsp chopped fresh mint	handful beansprouts
salt and pepper	handful salted peanuts
	1 red chilli (optional)
	2 x 170g/6oz sirloin steaks
	1 tbsp olive oil

1 To make the dressing, whisk the dressing ingredients together and season to taste (you won't need salt if using the tamari sauce).

2 Finely slice the pepper and spring onions and cut the cucumber into matchstick pieces. Peel the carrot and, using a potato peeler, continue to pare the carrot into slivers.

3 Place the salad leaves in two individual salad bowls and then add the pepper, spring onion, cucumber, carrot, beansprouts and peanuts, saving a few peanuts as a garnish. Finely dice the red chilli and save this also as a garnish.

4 Pat the steaks dry with kitchen paper, then smear both sides with olive oil. Fry the steaks over a medium to high heat until seared on both sides, then turn the heat to medium and cook for approximately 8 minutes, turning regularly until the steaks are cooked but still a little pink in the middle.

5 Discard any fat and cut the steaks into 1cm/½in strips. Pile onto the salads while still warm, pour over the dressing and garnish with the chilli and peanuts. Serve at once.

Duck and Orange Salad
with Beansprouts and Watercress

Serves 2

This recipe produces a simple but unforgettable salad with a zesty dressing. To speed up the cooking process, cut the duck breasts into bite-sized pieces.

salad leaves (to include watercress)	2.5cm/1in piece ginger
2 oranges	coriander leaves to garnish
2 handfuls beansprouts	
4 tbsp cooked fresh or frozen peas	DRESSING:
10cm/4in piece cucumber	90ml/3fl oz orange juice
2 spring onions	3 tbsp olive oil
2 duck breasts	1 tbsp fish sauce (optional)
1 tbsp olive oil	1 level tsp mustard
1 garlic clove	salt and pepper

1   Line two individual salad bowls with the salad leaves.
2   Peel and segment the oranges. Squeeze the membrane and a few segments to produce the orange juice for the dressing.
3   Place the remaining orange segments on the salad leaves, along with the beansprouts and peas. Cut the cucumber into dice and finely slice the spring onions and add these to the salads.
4   Skin and dry the duck breasts on kitchen paper. Press the garlic clove and grate the ginger then sweat these and the duck breasts in the olive oil until just cooked. Transfer the duck breasts onto a cutting board.
5   Slice the duck breasts into 1cm/½in slices, returning any juices that escape to the pan.
6   Add the dressing ingredients to the pan and mix with the juices. Season to taste with salt and pepper (you won't need salt if using the fish sauce).
7   Scatter the duck slices over the salads and drizzle over the dressing. Garnish with coriander leaves and serve at once.

Smoked Salmon, Prawn and Avocado Salad
Serves 2

This salad combination has stood the test of time. It is still irresistible and is one of my favourites.

	DRESSING:
mixed salad leaves	6 tbsp soya or other yogurt
1 large avocado	1 level tsp mustard
8 cherry tomatoes	1 tbsp tomato purée
7.5cm/3in piece cucumber	1 tbsp lemon juice
2 spring onions	1 tsp honey (optional)
4 slices smoked salmon	salt and pepper
225g/8oz cooked prawns	

1 Place the salad leaves in two individual salad bowls.
2 Peel the avocado, remove the stone and cut the flesh into bite-sized pieces.
3 Cut the cherry tomatoes in half and the cucumber into dice, and finely slice the spring onions.
4 Cut the smoked salmon into strips and scatter on top of the salad leaves along with the avocado, tomatoes, cucumber, spring onions and prawns. Save a few pieces as a garnish.
5 To make the dressing, whisk together the yogurt, mustard, tomato purée, lemon juice and honey. Season to taste with salt and pepper and drizzle the dressing over the salads.
6 Garnish with the reserved ingredients and serve at once.

Meat Dishes

Duck Breasts with Orange, Ginger and Sage

Serves 2

Duck and orange are the perfect partners. Here, cooked with ginger and sage, their contrasting colours, textures and flavours make a delightful meal.

2 duck breasts	140ml/5fl oz stock
1 tbsp olive oil	8 sage leaves, fresh or dried
2 medium onions	1 heaped tsp corn or rice flour
1 garlic clove	140ml/5fl oz orange juice
2.5cm/1in piece ginger	salt and pepper
1 small orange	parsley to garnish

1 Skin the duck breasts and dry on kitchen paper.
2 Heat the oil in a large frying pan over a medium heat and add the duck breasts. Fry gently for a few minutes to seal the meat on both sides.
3 Cut the onions into wedges, press the garlic clove, grate the ginger and add them to the frying pan. Sweat the ingredients until the onions are starting to soften and brown.
4 Cut the orange into slices and add to the pan along with the stock and sage leaves. Bring to the boil and cover with a loose-fitting lid. Simmer for approximately 10 minutes or until the duck and onions are cooked.
5 Combine the flour and orange juice and add to the pan. Bring to the boil, stirring constantly, and simmer for 2 minutes.
6 Season to taste with salt and pepper and, if you prefer, remove the sage leaves. Garnish with parsley and serve with rice, millet or quinoa.

Duck Breasts with Ginger, Garlic and Spring Onions

Serves 2

This dish is so easy to prepare yet it produces a meal that is special enough for any occasion. To speed up the cooking process still further, dice the duck breasts before cooking.

1 garlic clove	2 duck breasts
1cm/½in piece ginger	1 dsp tamari sauce (optional)
1 bunch spring onions	salt and pepper
1 tbsp olive oil	

1   Press the garlic clove, finely slice the ginger and cut the spring onions into chunks.
2   Heat the oil in a pan and lightly fry the duck breasts on both sides. Add the ginger, garlic and spring onions, turn the heat down to low, cover the ingredients with a loose-fitting lid and sweat them until cooked. This will take approximately 10 minutes, depending on the thickness of the duck and how well you like it cooked.
3   Lift the duck breasts from the pan onto serving plates and add the tamari sauce to the pan, if using this. Stir to combine and season to taste with salt and pepper (you won't need salt if using tamari sauce).
4   Pile the garlic, ginger and spring onions over the duck breasts and serve with vegetables or salad.

Ginger, Peach and Chicken Stir-Fry
Serves 2

Stir-frying is the perfect way to make a delicious, colourful and speedy meal. Use mango when fresh peach is not in season. You can also use other vegetables instead of mangetout – try courgettes and peppers. Water chestnuts are available in tins in most supermarkets and add a lovely crunch to this recipe.

2 chicken breasts	½ tsp dried dill or 1 dsp fresh
2 small peaches	1 rounded tsp corn or rice flour
6 spring onions	115g/4oz mangetout
2.5cm/1in piece ginger	14 water chestnuts
1 tbsp olive oil	salt and pepper
240ml/8fl oz stock	chopped parsley to garnish
¼ tsp cinnamon	

1   Cut the chicken breasts into bite-sized pieces. Peel and stone the peaches and cut into chunks. Slice the spring onions into 2cm/¾in lengths and grate the ginger.
2   Sweat the chicken, spring onions and ginger in the olive oil until the chicken is beginning to colour and the onions soften.
3   Mix the stock with the cinnamon, dill and flour and add this to the pan along with the mangetout and water chestnuts.
4   Bring to the boil, stirring continuously, and simmer for approximately 5 minutes or until the vegetables and chicken are tender.
5   Add the peaches and heat through. Season the stir-fry to taste with salt and pepper, garnish with parsley and serve with rice, millet or quinoa.

Chicken with Lime and Tarragon
Serves 2

This is a simple and exceedingly tasty way of serving chicken. Use lemon juice if you do not have a lime. If you want to serve the chicken breasts whole, follow the recipe up to step 3, then add the stock and simmer for 10–15 minutes until the chicken breasts are cooked. Remove the chicken breasts from the pan, add the lime and tarragon – and a little more liquid if the stock has evaporated – then bring to the boil, add the soya yogurt and heat through. Season and serve the sauce poured over the chicken breasts.

2 chicken breasts	1 dsp lime juice
1 onion	1 tsp grated lime rind
1 garlic clove	2 tbsp chopped fresh tarragon
1 tbsp olive oil	6 tbsp soya yogurt
90ml/3fl oz chicken stock	salt and pepper

1 Cut the chicken breasts into bite-sized pieces, dice the onion and press the garlic clove.
2 Sweat the chicken, onion and garlic in the olive oil until the chicken is almost cooked and beginning to brown.
3 Add the stock, lime juice, lime rind and tarragon (saving a little as a garnish). Bring to the boil and simmer for approximately 5 minutes or until the chicken is fully cooked.
4 Add the soya yogurt and bring to the boil but do not continue to cook as the yogurt may start to separate. Season to taste with salt and pepper and garnish with the remaining tarragon. This dish is delicious served with rice and a green salad.

Chicken with Basil, Spring Onions and Pickled Lemon

Serves 2

To make this recipe quick and easy, I cut the chicken into pieces and serve it in the sauce, but the chicken breasts could be griddled and the sauce served alongside. To make the sauce separately, sweat the garlic and spring onions and, when cooked, add the basil, pickled lemon, stock and the butter or margarine. Heat through and pour over the chicken.

2 chicken breasts	2 heaped tbsp chopped fresh basil
1 garlic clove	1 tbsp finely chopped pickled lemon
1 tbsp olive oil	1 tbsp butter or margarine
1 bunch spring onions	salt and pepper
60ml/2fl oz stock	

1　Cut the chicken into bite-sized pieces and press the garlic clove. Sweat the chicken and garlic in the olive oil until the meat is nearly cooked.

2　Cut the spring onions into chunks and add to the pan along with the stock. Bring to the boil and simmer for approximately 5 minutes or until the chicken and spring onions are both cooked.

3　Add the basil, pickled lemon and the butter or margarine. Bring to the boil and season to taste with salt and pepper.

4　Serve with potatoes, pasta or rice and vegetables or salad.

Tamarind and Chilli Chicken

Serves 2

Sometimes when I'm inventing recipes I get a name in my head first, then go on to produce the recipe. When I came to type up the recipes for this book, I found I'd created two recipes for tamarind and chilli chicken and both had worked well, so here they are. Tamarind gives this spicy dish a delicious tangy lemon flavour.

1 bunch spring onions	1 rounded tsp tamarind paste
2 chicken breasts	140ml/5fl oz stock
1 large garlic clove	1 tsp corn or rice flour
1 red chilli	salt and pepper
1 tbsp olive oil	roasted peanuts or coriander leaves to
½ tbsp fish sauce (optional)	garnish

1 Cut the spring onions into chunks and the chicken into bite-sized pieces. Press the garlic clove and deseed and finely dice the chilli.
2 Sweat the chicken, spring onions, garlic and chilli in the olive oil until the chicken begins to brown.
3 Whisk together the fish sauce, tamarind paste, stock and flour and add to the chicken mix in the pan. Bring to the boil and simmer for 10 minutes or until the chicken is cooked.
4 Season to taste with salt and pepper, garnish with roasted peanuts or coriander leaves and serve with rice.

Tamarind and Chilli Chicken II

Serves 2

This is another spicy meal that takes very little time to prepare and cook.

1 bunch spring onions	400g tin chopped tomatoes
2 chicken breasts	1 rounded tsp tamarind paste
1 large garlic clove	10 curry leaves
1 red chilli	salt and pepper
1 tbsp olive oil	1 tbsp chopped fresh coriander
1 level dsp ground coriander	

1 Cut the spring onions into chunks and the chicken into bite-sized pieces. Press the garlic clove and deseed and finely dice the chilli.
2 Sweat the chicken, spring onions, garlic and chilli in the olive oil until the chicken begins to brown.
3 Add the ground coriander and sweat the ingredients for a few more minutes.
4 Add the tomatoes, tamarind and the curry leaves, bring to the boil and simmer for approximately 10 minutes or until the chicken is cooked.
5 Remove the curry leaves and season to taste with salt and pepper. Garnish with the fresh coriander and serve with rice, millet or quinoa.

Moroccan Spiced Lemon Chicken
Serves 2

This easy-to-prepare dish is full of the robust flavours of Moroccan cooking. If you wish to serve this as a casserole, use chicken joints instead of breasts and cook it in the oven for an hour. Do not add the flour but mix this with a little cold water and add to the juices once cooked. Bring the casserole to the boil, simmer for 2 minutes then season and serve.

1 medium onion	½ tsp paprika
1 garlic clove	240ml/8fl oz stock or water
2.5cm/1in piece ginger	2 tbsp tomato purée (optional)
1 tbsp olive oil	2 tbsp finely chopped preserved lemon
2 chicken breasts	1 rounded tsp corn or rice flour
½ tsp cinnamon	salt and pepper
½ tsp turmeric	1 tbsp chopped fresh coriander
½ tsp cumin	

1 Dice the onion, press the garlic clove and finely grate the ginger. Sweat these in the olive oil until the onion begins to soften.
2 Cut the chicken breasts into bite-sized pieces and add to the pan along with the cinnamon, turmeric, cumin and paprika. Cook for 5 minutes, stirring occasionally.
3 Mix together the stock, tomato purée, preserved lemon and flour and pour over the chicken. Bring to the boil, stirring constantly, and simmer for 10 minutes or until the chicken is cooked.
4 Season to taste with salt and pepper and stir in the coriander. Serve with rice and salad or vegetables.

Chicken Satay Kebabs

Serves 2

If you want a change from chicken, you can use steak, lamb or duck breasts in this recipe. Ideally the meat should marinate for a few hours. If you like, you can also make the satay sauce in advance and warm it through before serving.

MARINADE:	SATAY SAUCE:
1 garlic clove	4 tbsp peanut butter
1 tsp olive oil	140ml/5fl oz coconut milk
1 tsp sesame oil	1 tbsp lemon juice
1 tbsp lemon juice	1 level tsp honey (optional)
1 tsp tamari sauce (optional)	1 tsp tamari sauce (optional)
⅛–¼ tsp chilli powder	1 pressed garlic clove
salt and pepper	salt and pepper
2 large chicken breasts	

1   First, make the marinade. Press the garlic clove and place in a bowl with the olive oil, sesame oil, lemon juice, tamari sauce, chilli powder and a little salt and pepper. Whisk to combine the marinade ingredients.
2   Cut the chicken breasts into bite-sized chunks, add to the marinade and set aside, preferably for a few hours but at least while you prepare the satay sauce.
3   To make the satay sauce, place all the ingredients in a pan and heat, stirring occasionally, until well combined. Season to taste with salt and pepper and keep warm.
4   Thread the chicken pieces onto two large or four small skewers, folding over the chicken where it is thinner so that the pieces are even sized.
5   Cook under a hot grill for approximately 5 minutes on each side or until the chicken is cooked. Baste during cooking with any remaining marinade.
6   Serve with rice, millet, quinoa or pasta, and a salad.

Chicken and Broccoli with Noodles

Serves 2

In this recipe, the chicken, vegetables and noodles sit in a soup-like sauce that is absolutely delicious. Use a spoon to eat it or mop up the juices with crusty bread, if acceptable. There are countless variations on this recipe – try other vegetables, add some prawns with the chicken or use duck or beef.

2 chicken breasts	1 tbsp tamari or fish sauce (optional)
1 bunch spring onions	4 kaffir lime leaves
5cm/2in piece ginger	½ red pepper
2 garlic cloves	1 small courgette
½–1 red chilli	225g/6oz broccoli
1 tbsp olive oil	250g/9oz buckwheat or rice noodles
285ml/10fl oz coconut milk	salt and pepper
425ml/15fl oz stock	1 tbsp chopped fresh coriander
1 tbsp lemon juice	

1 Cut the chicken breasts into bite-sized pieces and the spring onions into 2cm/1in lengths. Finely slice half the ginger and grate the rest. Press the garlic cloves and finely dice the chilli. Sweat all these ingredients in the olive oil until the chicken changes colour.

2 Add the coconut milk, stock, lemon juice, tamari or fish sauce and the kaffir lime leaves.

3 Cut the red pepper and courgette into slices and break the broccoli into florets. Add these to the pan with the noodles. Bring to the boil and simmer for approximately 10 minutes or until the chicken, vegetables and noodles are cooked. Remove the kaffir lime leaves and season to taste with salt and pepper. Serve in large bowls, garnished with the coriander.

Chicken, Pineapple and Red Pepper in a Sweet and Sour Sauce

Serves 2

This recipe is a colourful and irresistible combination of ingredients. Omit the tomato purée if you cannot tolerate tomatoes – the sauce will look a little pale but will taste fine. You can use duck breasts as an alternative to the chicken in this recipe.

2 chicken breasts	1 tbsp tomato purée
1 small red pepper	1 tbsp tamari sauce (optional)
1 medium onion	170g/6oz pineapple chunks (tinned or
1 garlic clove	fresh)
1 tbsp olive oil	salt and pepper
140ml/5fl oz pineapple juice	parsley to garnish
1 tsp corn or rice flour	

1 Cut the chicken into bite-sized pieces, slice the red pepper, dice the onion and press the garlic clove.
2 Sweat the chicken in the olive oil until it begins to brown. Add the garlic, peppers and onion and sweat these until they begin to soften.
3 Whisk together the pineapple juice, flour, tomato purée and tamari and add to the pan along with the pineapple chunks.
4 Bring to the boil, stirring, and simmer for a few more minutes until the vegetables and chicken are cooked.
5 Season to taste with salt and pepper. Garnish with parsley and serve with rice or noodles and a salad.

Sautéed Kidneys in a Creamy Sauce
Serves 2

If you can, buy organic kidneys for this recipe. Other vegetables can be used instead when you want a change from mushrooms and carrots – try courgettes, peppers and mangetout. If you cannot tolerate soya, try sheep, goat's or cow's milk yogurt. Omit the tomato purée if you cannot tolerate tomatoes.

6 lambs' kidneys	½ tsp dried rosemary
1 medium onion	½ tsp dried thyme
1 garlic clove	1 tbsp tomato purée
115g/4oz mushrooms	1 level tsp mustard
1 medium carrot	180g/6oz soya yogurt
1 tbsp olive oil	1 tbsp chopped fresh parsley

1 Remove the skin and core from the kidneys and cut into bite-sized pieces.
2 Dice the onion and press the garlic clove. Half or quarter the mushrooms depending on their size. Peel the carrot then cut it into ribbons using a peeler.
3 Sweat the onion, garlic and carrot in the oil until they are almost cooked. Add the kidneys, mushrooms and herbs and continue to sweat the ingredients until the kidneys and vegetables are just cooked. This will only take a few minutes.
4 Add the tomato purée, mustard and the yogurt and stir to combine. Bring to the boil but do not continue to cook or the yogurt may start to separate.
5 Garnish with parsley and serve with rice and salad.

Beef Stroganoff

Serves 2

This is such an impressive dish – easy and quick to make, scrumptious to eat and suitable for any occasion.

340g/12oz beef fillet	1 dsp paprika
1 onion	1 rounded tsp mustard powder
1 garlic clove	225g/8oz soya yogurt
225g/8oz chestnut mushrooms	1 tbsp chopped fresh parsley
1 tbsp olive oil	salt and pepper

1 Cut the beef into slices 1cm/½in thick, then cut each slice across the grain into thin strips. Thinly slice the onion, press the garlic clove and cut the mushrooms into quarters.

2 Sweat the onion and garlic in the olive oil until the onion begins to soften. Toss the steak in the paprika and mustard then add to the pan along with the mushrooms. Continue to sweat until the steak is just cooked and the mushrooms are softened.

3 Add the soya yogurt and most of the parsley. Bring to the boil but do not continue to cook or the yogurt may begin to separate.

4 Season to taste with salt and pepper and serve on rice, garnished with the remaining parsley.

Thai Green Curry Paste

Doesn't it sound complicated making your own green curry paste? Well it isn't, in fact it couldn't be simpler. I find ready-made curry pastes so hot that I can only use a little and, as a result, my curry ends up with a lot of heat but not much flavour. Personally, I prefer more flavour and not too much heat. (If you wish, you can use a ready-made paste, as most contain acceptable ingredients, but follow the manufacturer's suggestions as to the quantity to use.) The ingredients below make sufficient paste for two or three curries but I usually double or treble the quantities and freeze the paste in ice cube trays for future use. Vegetarians can omit the fish sauce and add 1 tablespoon of tamari sauce if this is acceptable.

2 shallots	1 tsp grated lemon rind
2 garlic cloves	1 tbsp fish sauce (optional)
5cm/2in piece fresh ginger	2 tbsp olive oil
1 stalk lemon grass	1 rounded tsp ground coriander
½–1 green chilli (more if you want a hot curry)	½ tsp ground cumin
	2 tbsp chopped fresh coriander
2 tbsp lemon or lime juice	¼ tsp salt

1 Peel the shallots, garlic and ginger and the outer tough leaves from the lemon grass. De-seed the chilli.
2 If you have a good food processor then literally throw all the ingredients in and whiz until you have a fairly smooth paste. If you feel your machine may struggle then give it a bit of help by pressing the garlic, grating the ginger and finely slicing the lemon grass, shallots and chilli.
3 Store the paste in the fridge and use within a week or freeze.

Thai Chicken Curry

Serves 2

You can vary this curry by substituting coconut milk or chopped tomatoes for the soya yogurt, coriander for the basil leaves and beef or lamb for the chicken. You could also add a few vegetables with the meat for a meat and vegetable curry – try broccoli, onions, mangetout, baby sweetcorn and courgette.

2 large chicken breasts	285g/10oz soya yogurt
1 tbsp olive oil	2 tbsp chopped fresh basil leaves
2 heaped tbsp Thai Green Curry Paste (see page 106)	salt and pepper

1 Cut the chicken breasts into bite-sized pieces and sweat the meat in the olive oil until it begins to brown.
2 Add the curry paste and continue to sweat the chicken until it is just cooked.
3 Add the soya yogurt and most of the basil leaves, saving a few chopped leaves as a garnish. Bring to the boil, but do not over-cook or the yogurt may separate. Season to taste with salt and pepper, garnish with the basil and serve with cooked rice, millet or quinoa.

Thai Lamb and Vegetable Curry
Serves 2

The flavours of the East shine through in this exceedingly tasty curry. Other vegetables could be substituted for the onion and carrot, such as parsnips and leeks, and you could add tinned tomatoes instead of the stock or water. If you wish, miss out the sweating for an even quicker curry – the flavour will still be quite acceptable.

1 onion	455g/1lb lean stewing lamb
1 carrot	240ml/8fl oz stock or water
1 red pepper	½ tbsp tamari sauce (optional)
1 tbsp olive oil	240ml/8fl oz coconut milk
3 heaped tbsp Thai Green Curry Paste	2 tbsp chopped fresh coriander
(see page 106)	salt and pepper

1 Set the oven temperature to 190°C/375°F/Gas Mark 5.
2 Roughly chop the onion, carrot and red pepper and sweat these in the olive oil, in a casserole dish, until they begin to soften and brown.
3 Add the curry paste and cook for a few minutes.
4 Add the lamb, water or stock, tamari sauce and coconut milk.
5 Cover the casserole dish and cook in the oven for 1¾ hours or until the lamb is tender.
6 Mix in most of the coriander, saving a little as a garnish, and season to taste with salt and pepper. Garnish with coriander and serve with rice.

Spiced One-Pot Chicken
Serves 2

This is a simple way of cooking chicken and vegetables together. While the oven is on why not throw in some baking potatoes so that your meal is complete?

900g/2lb selection of vegetables e.g. butternut squash, shallots, carrots, peppers, parsnips, fennel, celery 3 tbsp Thai Green Curry Paste (see page 106)	140ml/5fl oz orange juice 2 chicken leg portions 1 tsp olive oil parsley or coriander to garnish

1 Set the oven temperature to 200°C/400°F/Gas Mark 6.
2 Cut the vegetables into large chunks that will cook in roughly the same time. Place in an ovenproof dish that is big enough to hold the vegetables in a single layer.
3 Mix together the curry paste and orange juice and pour over the vegetables. Mix well so that all the vegetables are coated.
4 Rub the olive oil into the chicken skins and place the portions on top of the vegetables.
5 Bake in the oven, uncovered, for approximately 1 hour, basting the vegetables and chicken occasionally with the marinade.
6 Garnish with the parsley or coriander and serve with baked potatoes or rice.

Mediterranean Chicken
with Olives and Peppers

Serves 2

The flavours of the Mediterranean dominate this delicious dish. While it cooks in the oven, why not add some baking potatoes so that you can have an hour off as the meal cooks? This is another dish where the vegetables can be sweated first in olive oil for extra flavour, though it's fine without this and certainly easier.

1 onion	10 black olives
1 garlic clove	2 sun-dried tomatoes
½ red pepper	1 small orange
1 large courgette	2 chicken leg portions
400g tin chopped tomatoes	1 tsp olive oil
240ml/8fl oz stock or water	1 rounded tsp corn or rice flour
1 tsp dried basil	salt and pepper
1 tsp dried oregano	parsley to garnish

1   Set the oven temperature to 200°C/400°F/Gas Mark 6.

2   Dice the onion, press the garlic clove and slice the pepper and courgette. Place these in a casserole dish.

3   Add the tomatoes, stock or water, basil, oregano and the olives.

4   Finely dice the sun-dried tomatoes and cut the unpeeled orange into wedges. Add those to the casserole dish, saving a few orange wedges as a garnish. Stir to combine.

5   Place the chicken joints on top of the casserole and, using your fingers, smear the olive oil over the chicken skin. Bake, uncovered, for 1 hour or until the chicken is cooked. If the chicken is browning too quickly, cover the dish loosely with foil.

6   Remove the chicken. To thicken the juices, mix the flour with a little water and add to the casserole. Bring to the boil on the hob and simmer for 1 minute. Season to taste with salt and pepper.

7   Garnish the chicken and vegetables with the parsley and the orange wedges and serve with rice, pasta or baked potatoes.

Baked Chicken with Herby Rice

Serves 2

The art to successfully making this dish lies in ensuring the rice is just cooked and fluffy as all the stock is absorbed. As different types of rice soak up different amounts of liquid, and oven temperatures vary, you'll need to keep an eye on the casserole the first time you make it. Add a little extra stock or lengthen the cooking time if necessary. After that it's a cinch to cook.

1 medium onion	1 bay leaf
2 medium carrots	710ml/1¼ pints stock
1 medium parsnip	1 tsp olive oil
200g/7oz brown basmati rice	2 chicken leg joints
½ tsp dried rosemary	salt and pepper
½ tsp dried thyme	1 tbsp chopped fresh parsley

1 Set the oven temperature to 200°C/400°F/Gas Mark 6.
2 Cut the onion, carrots and parsnip into bite-sized pieces and place these in a deep casserole dish.
3 Wash the brown rice well and add this to the casserole along with the rosemary, thyme, bay leaf and stock. Mix the ingredients to combine.
4 Rub the olive oil into skin of the chicken and place the legs on top of the rice and vegetables in the casserole dish.
5 Bake, uncovered, for 1 hour, by which time the chicken should be cooked and the rice should be fluffy and have absorbed all the stock.
6 Mix the parsley into the rice and, if necessary, season with salt and pepper. Serve the chicken and vegetables on top of the rice.

Chicken Risotto

Serves 2

It can be very time consuming to make a proper risotto. This is a cheat's version – it takes a fraction of the time yet it is equally delicious. I often make this if I have leftover cooked chicken, which I add along with the rice, just to heat it through. As an alternative to the vegetables listed below, you could try sweetcorn, mangetout, peppers and celery.

1 onion	455g/1lb slightly undercooked rice
1 garlic clove	(225g/8oz before cooking)
1 large courgette	240ml/8fl oz stock
115g/4oz mushrooms	1 tbsp chopped parsley
1 chicken breast (approx. 170g/6oz)	½ tbsp tamari sauce (optional)
1 tbsp olive oil	salt and pepper
	parsley to garnish

1 Dice the onion, press the garlic clove, slice the courgette and quarter the mushrooms. Cut the chicken into small pieces.

2 Sweat the onion and garlic in the olive oil until the onion just starts to soften. Add the courgette and chicken and continue to cook for approximately 5 minutes. Finally, add the mushrooms and allow them to soften.

3 Add the rice, stock, parsley and tamari sauce. Bring to the boil and simmer, stirring occasionally, until everything is well cooked and most of the stock has been absorbed.

4 Season to taste with salt and pepper and serve in pasta or salad bowls, garnished with parsley.

Lamb Hot-Pot

Serves 2

What could be nicer on a cold winter's day than a hot-pot of meat and vegetables bubbling away in the oven and a wonderful aroma pervading the home? For extra flavour, you could sweat the meat and vegetables in olive oil but I've missed out this stage to save time.

455g/1lb lean lamb	½ tsp rosemary
1 rounded tbsp corn or rice flour	1 level tsp mustard
1 onion	285ml/½ pint stock
1 carrot	salt and pepper
1 stick celery	680g/1½lb potatoes
1 bay leaf	1 tbsp olive oil
½ tsp thyme	

1   Set the oven temperature to 190°C/375°F/Gas Mark 5.
2   Cube the lamb and toss in the flour to coat.
3   Cut the onion into wedges, the carrot into chunks and slice the celery.
4   Place the meat, vegetables, bay leaf, thyme, rosemary, mustard and stock in a casserole dish and stir to combine. Season the hot-pot with salt and pepper.
5   Peel the potatoes and cut into dice approximately 1½cm/¾in square. Dry these on kitchen paper or a clean tea towel and place in a bowl with the olive oil. Stir to coat the potatoes with the oil.
6   Pile the potatoes on top of the meat and vegetables and spread out to cover the surface.
7   Bake the hot-pot, uncovered, for 2 hours. When cooked, the potatoes should be brown and crisp on top. If they are browning too quickly, cover loosely with some foil. Serve in bowls and eat with spoons. Whoever finds the bay leaf can fish it out.

Hungarian-Style Goulash
Serves 2

This is another dish that is left to bubble away in the oven while you get on with other things. It has a wonderful combination of flavours and textures and goes well with simply cooked vegetables or salads. For extra flavour, sweat the vegetables and meat in a tablespoon of olive oil before adding to the casserole dish. Substitute lamb for the beef if you prefer.

1 large onion	285ml/10fl oz stock or water
1 garlic clove	1 tbsp tomato purée (optional)
455g/1lb lean stewing beef	2 medium potatoes
1 level tbsp smoked paprika	salt and pepper
1 level tsp caraway seeds	140g/5oz soya or other yogurt
1 tsp dried oregano	1 tbsp chopped fresh parsley
400g tin chopped tomatoes	

1 Set the oven temperature to 200°C/400°F/Gas Mark 6.
2 Cut the onion into chunks and press the garlic clove.
3 Place the onion and garlic in a casserole dish with the meat, paprika, caraway seeds, oregano, chopped tomatoes, stock and the tomato purée. Stir well to combine and cover the casserole.
4 Cook the casserole for 30 minutes in the oven. Roughly chop the potatoes and add these to the casserole dish. Cook for 1 hour or until the potatoes and meat are both tender.
5 Season to taste with salt and pepper, then swirl the yogurt through the goulash. Garnish with parsley and serve.

Lamb Tagine with Apricots and Almonds
Serves 2

This gorgeous combination of meat, fruit, spices and nuts is typical of the
exceedingly tasty cuisine of north Africa. For a variation on this tagine,
substitute beef for the lamb and prunes for the apricots. Fresh ginger
makes a good addition and butterbeans could be used instead of the
almonds. For extra flavour, the lamb and vegetables can be sweated in a
little oil before adding to the casserole. If you cannot tolerate tomatoes just
add extra stock instead; if you cannot tolerate citrus omit the lemon.

455g/1lb lean stewing lamb	12 whole almonds
1 tsp turmeric	400g tin chopped tomatoes
1 tsp paprika	240ml/8fl oz stock or water
1 tsp cinnamon	1 tbsp chopped pickled lemon
1 large onion	salt and pepper
1 garlic clove	1 tbsp chopped fresh coriander
8 dried apricots	

1 Set the oven temperature to 190°C/375°F/Gas Mark 5.
2 Cube the lamb and place in a casserole dish. Add the turmeric, paprika
   and cinnamon and toss to coat the lamb.
3 Cut the onion into chunks and press the garlic clove. Add to the casserole,
   along with the apricots, almonds, tomatoes and stock.
4 Mix to combine, cover the casserole and cook in the oven for approximately 2 hours, by which time the lamb should be tender and sitting in a
   thick sauce. If the sauce is not thick enough, evaporate a little of the liquid
   by cooking the casserole, uncovered, on a higher heat.
5 Add the pickled lemon and season to taste with salt and pepper. Garnish
   with the coriander and serve with rice, noodles or baked potatoes.

Butternut Squash and Spiced Lamb Stew

Serves 2

I love to make winter casseroles when autumn vegetables come into the shops. This hearty, warming stew is satisfying and full of robust flavours.

455g/1lb butternut squash	140ml/5fl oz apple or orange juice
2.5cm/1in piece ginger	115g/4oz baby spinach
2 garlic cloves	salt and pepper
340g/12oz lean stewing lamb	140g/5oz soya or other yogurt
1 tsp caraway seeds	handful fresh coriander leaves
1 tsp fennel or cumin seeds	

1　Set the oven temperature to 180°C/350°F/Gas Mark 4.
2　Remove the seeds from the butternut squash and the skin if it is blemished or tough. Cube the flesh.
3　Finely slice the ginger, press the garlic clove and cut the lamb into even-sized cubes.
4　Place the ginger, garlic and lamb in a casserole dish with the squash, caraway seeds, fennel or cumin seeds, and the fruit juice.
5　Cover the casserole and cook for 1¼ hours. Remove the casserole from the oven, stir well with a wooden spoon and break up some of the butternut squash. Add the spinach and cook for another 30 minutes.
6　Season to taste with salt and pepper and swirl in the yogurt and coriander before serving.

Venison Casserole

Serves 2

In winter, I love to put casseroles in the oven with baking potatoes and set the timer. There is nothing nicer on a cold day than to return home to the wonderful aroma of dinner cooking. Lamb or beef can be used instead of the venison in this recipe. Bottled horseradish is available with acceptable ingredients. I found one in a supermarket called 'hot horseradish', or see the list of suppliers at the back of this book.

455g/1lb stewing venison	1 tbsp chopped fresh thyme or 1 tsp
1 large onion	dried thyme
1 garlic clove	340ml/12fl oz stock or water
170g/6oz field mushrooms	1 bay leaf
1 tbsp bottled horseradish or 2 tbsp	1 level dsp corn or rice flour
fresh grated horseradish	salt and pepper
1 tbsp tomato purée (optional)	parsley to garnish

1   Set the oven temperature to 180°C/350°F/Gas Mark 4.
2   Dice the meat, cut the onion into chunks, press the garlic clove and quarter the mushrooms. Place these in a casserole dish.
3   Mix the horseradish, tomato purée and thyme with the stock or water and pour over the other ingredients in the casserole dish.
4   Add the bay leaf, cover the casserole and cook for 2 hours.
5   To thicken the casserole, mix the flour with a little water and stir this into the casserole. Bring to the boil on the hob and simmer for 2 minutes. Season the casserole to taste with salt and pepper and remove the bay leaf.
6   Garnish with parsley and serve with baked potatoes, rice or noodles, and with vegetables or salad.

Fish Dishes

Salmon with Green Lentils and Vegetables

Serves 2

This delicious, colourful and very speedy meal uses vegetables that take the same time to cook as the salmon. If you want to include vegetables that take longer, such as carrots, then part-cook them before you add the salmon. If you wish to use dried lentils, cook 115g/4oz in 570ml/1 pint of stock until soft

400g tin lentils	2 salmon fillets
340g/12oz selection of vegetables e.g. courgettes, mushrooms, mangetout, baby sweetcorn, spinach, fresh or frozen peas, fresh or frozen broad beans, peppers	lemon wedges and parsley to garnish

1 Place the lentils and their juices in a large frying pan.
2 Cut your chosen vegetables, where necessary, into pieces that will all cook in a similar amount of time.
3 Place these on top of the lentils.
4 Lay the salmon fillets on the vegetables, skin side uppermost and bring the mixture to the boil. Cover with a loose fitting lid and simmer for 8–10 minutes or until the salmon and vegetables are just cooked. The length of time required will depend on the thickness of the salmon.
5 Place the lentil and vegetable mixture in pasta bowls, put the salmon on top and garnish with the lemon wedges and parsley.

Fried Fish with Tomato and Pickled Lemon Salsa

Serves 2

Coating the fish in corn flour gives it a lovely golden colour but you could use other flours if you cannot tolerate corn. Salsas are very easy to make with any moist fruit and vegetables – try substituting avocado for the tomato or pineapple for the lemon.

2 tbsp corn flour	2 large ripe tomatoes
salt and pepper	2 dsp finely chopped pickled lemon
2 pieces white fish e.g. haddock,	1 tbsp chopped fresh herbs e.g.
hake, cod	coriander, parsley
3 tbsp olive oil	

1 Place the corn flour on a plate and season with salt and pepper.
2 Wash the fish and dry lightly with kitchen paper. Dip the fish into the seasoned corn flour until coated on both sides.
3 Fry the fish in 1 tablespoon of olive oil, over a medium heat, for approximately 5 minutes on each side or until just cooked. The length of time required will depend on the thickness of the fish.
4 To make the salsa, skin the tomatoes (place in boiling water for a few seconds to loosen the skins) and dice the flesh as finely as possible. Mix the tomatoes with the pickled lemon, fresh herbs and the two remaining tablespoons of olive oil.
5 Season the salsa to taste with salt and pepper and serve with the fish.

Fried Fish with Mango and Ginger Salsa

Serves 2

Fish has an affinity with the sharpness of fresh fruit, which is why it is often served with lemon. In this recipe, mango provides the tangy flavour. Look for a mango that is slightly under-ripe or it will be a little sweet. You can also substitute other fruit in this salsa, such as plums.

2 tbsp corn flour	½ small mango
salt and pepper	½ shallot
2 pieces white fish e.g. haddock,	1 tsp grated fresh ginger
hake, cod	1 dsp chopped fresh coriander
3 tbsp olive oil	1 dsp lemon juice (optional)

1 Place the corn flour on a plate and season it with salt and pepper.
2 Wash the fish and dry lightly with kitchen paper. Toss the fish in the corn flour until coated on both sides.
3 Fry the fish gently in 1 tablespoon of olive oil for approximately 5 minutes on each side until just cooked. The length of time required will depend on the thickness of the fish.
4 Dice the mango flesh and the shallot as finely as you can. Mix these with the grated ginger, chopped coriander, lemon juice and 2 tablespoons of olive oil.
5 Season the salsa to taste with salt and pepper and serve with the fish.

Baked Fish with Lemon and Herb Butter
Serves 2

I love meals where I can pop everything in the oven, and this fish dish fits the bill perfectly if you serve it with chips (see page 151) or roasted vegetables. You could substitute other herbs for the parsley in this recipe – try coriander, chives, fennel, basil, tarragon or a mixture of more than one.

2 thick pieces fresh white fish e.g. cod, haddock, hake, halibut	2 tbsp lemon juice
2 tbsp chopped fresh parsley	1 tbsp butter or margarine
½ level tsp mustard	salt and pepper

1 Set the oven temperature to 200°C/400°F/Gas Mark 6.
2 Place each piece of fish in the centre of a 30cm/12in square piece of foil.
3 Mix the chopped parsley with the mustard and lemon juice. Spread this mixture on the top of the two pieces of fish.
4 Dot the butter or margarine over the surface of the fish and season with salt and pepper. Draw up the corners of the foil to make two sealed parcels and place in the oven to bake for approximately 10–15 minutes (the time required will depend on the thickness of the fish).
5 Place the foil parcels onto serving plates and allow each person to open their own.

Grilled Salmon with Ginger, Garlic and Coriander
Serves 2

Fresh ginger and coriander combine in this recipe to give the salmon an unusual, piquant flavour. Because the fish is grilled it's best to use pieces that are not too thick – tail ends are ideal. Alternatively, use steaks and bake them in the oven for 10–15 minutes at 200°C/400°F/Gas Mark 6. You can also use other fish in this recipe, such as cod, haddock or plaice.

2 salmon fillets	1 tbsp olive oil
1 garlic clove	1 tbsp lemon juice
2.5cm/1in piece ginger	salt and pepper
1 tbsp chopped fresh coriander	

1 Line a baking tray with foil (this saves on washing up). Dry the fish and place it on the foil.
2 Press the garlic clove, finely grate the ginger and combine these with the coriander, olive oil and lemon juice. Spread this over the surface of the fish.
3 Season with salt and pepper.
4 Grill the fish on full power for approximately 10 minutes. The length of time required will depend on the thickness of the fish. Baste the fish with the juices while it is cooking and turn down the heat if the fish is browning too quickly.
5 Serve immediately with salad or cooked vegetables.

Grilled Fish with Tarragon and Pickled Lemon

Serves 2

As the fish in this recipe is grilled it's best to use tail ends, which are not too thick. If you wish to use fish steaks, bake them in the oven, uncovered, for approximately 10–15 minutes at 200°C/400°F/Gas Mark 6. Pickled lemons are now readily available in supermarkets and are worth seeking out as they add a special touch to this dish. Alternatively, use a teaspoon of grated lemon rind.

2 pieces fish e.g. salmon, cod, haddock, hake	1 tbsp finely chopped pickled lemon
	1 tbsp olive oil
2 tbsp chopped fresh tarragon	salt and pepper

1 Line a baking tray with foil (this saves on washing up). Dry the fish and place it on the foil.
2 Mix the tarragon, pickled lemon and olive oil and spread over the fish.
3 Season with salt and pepper.
4 Grill the fish on full power for approximately 10 minutes. The length of time required will depend on the thickness of the fish. Baste the fish occasionally with the juices while it is cooking. Turn the heat down a little if the surface is browning too quickly.
5 Serve immediately with salad or cooked vegetables.

Mediterranean-Style Baked Fish with Vegetables

Serves 2

This is a sublime combination of baked fish, herby roasted vegetables and basil-flavoured tomatoes. Courgette or aubergine could be added instead of the potatoes or peppers, and chopped anchovies could be used instead of black olives. The tomatoes can be omitted and the fish brushed with olive oil to bake.

565g/1¼lb waxy new potatoes	55g/2oz pitted black olives
1 large red onion	2 thick-cut pieces fish e.g. tuna,
1 red pepper	salmon, swordfish, cod
1 yellow pepper	½ x 400g tin chopped tomatoes
2 garlic cloves	2 tbsp chopped fresh basil
1 dsp chopped fresh thyme	Basil leaves to garnish
2 tbsp olive oil	

1 Set the oven temperature to 200°C/400°F/Gas 6.
2 Cut the potatoes into bite-sized pieces, the onion into 6 pieces and the peppers into quarters. Press the garlic cloves and toss these, the thyme and the vegetables in the olive oil.
3 Place the vegetables on a baking tray and cook, uncovered, for approximately 30 minutes or until the vegetables begin to soften and turn golden.
4 Place the vegetables in a shallow ovenproof baking dish and mix in the black olives. Place the fish pieces on top of the vegetables.
5 Mix the basil and chopped tomatoes and pour over the fish.
6 Bake for another 15 minutes or until the fish is just cooked. Serve immediately, garnished with a few basil leaves and with some green salad if desired.

Sardine and Potato Curry
Serves 2

Don't be put off by the idea of a fish curry – this one works really well and is very easy to prepare. I often make this with leftover cooked potatoes, in which case I only add 140ml/5fl oz of boiling water.

1 large onion	120g tin sardines in water or olive oil
1 tbsp olive oil	1 dsp fish sauce (optional)
3 tbsp Thai Green Curry Paste (see page 106)	140ml/5fl oz coconut milk
	1 tbsp chopped fresh coriander
455g/1lb new potatoes	salt and pepper
285ml/½ pint boiling water	coriander leaves to garnish

1 Dice the onion and sweat it in the olive oil until it begins to soften.
2 Add the curry paste and cook for a few minutes.
3 Cut the new potatoes into bite-sized pieces and add to the pan along with the water. Bring to the boil and simmer until the potatoes are just cooked.
4 Drain the sardines, remove the bones and cut the flesh into small pieces. Add to the pan along with the fish sauce, coconut milk and coriander.
5 Heat through and season to taste if necessary (you won't need salt if using the fish sauce).
6 Garnish with coriander leaves and serve with rice.

Speedy Tuna and Tomato Pasta
Serves 2

This really is instant food so it's great when you're in a hurry. If you use a tin of chopped tomatoes with basil you can miss out the fresh herbs. If you want to make this dish a little more elaborate add vegetables such as courgettes, mushrooms, peppers and onions, preferably sweated in a little olive oil until they are soft. If using wheat pasta, you won't need to use as much – 170g/6oz should be sufficient.

225g/8oz rice pasta
400g tin chopped tomatoes
185g tin tuna in water or olive oil

2 tbsp fresh or frozen herbs e.g. basil, coriander, parsley

1 Cook the pasta according to the manufacturer's instructions and drain.
2 Return the pasta to the pan and add the chopped tomatoes, drained tuna and the herbs.
3 Bring to the boil, simmer for 5 minutes and serve.

Sardine, Olive and Tomato Pasta

Use a 120g tin of sardines instead of the tuna used in the above recipe, and add about 10 halved olives.

cooking without made easy

Poached Fish with Ginger and Spring Onions
Serves 2

This dish can also be baked in the oven, in foil parcels, at 200°C/ 400°F/Gas Mark 6. If you decide to do this, don't sweat the vegetables but mix these with the olive oil, pile them on top of the fish and omit the stock or water. Bake for approximately 15 minutes.

1cm/½in piece ginger	60ml/2fl oz stock or water
1 garlic clove	2 pieces fish e.g. cod, haddock,
1 bunch spring onions	swordfish, hake, halibut
1 tbsp olive oil	salt and pepper

1 Grate the ginger, press the garlic clove and finely slice the spring onions. Sweat these in the olive oil for a few minutes until the onions begin to soften a little.
2 Add the stock or water and place the fish on top. Cover loosely with a lid and simmer for approximately 10–15 minutes until the fish is cooked. The time required will depend on the thickness of the fish.
3 Remove the fish and place on serving plates. Season the juices with salt and pepper and pour over the fish.
4 Serve with salad or vegetables.

Monkfish and Prawn Provençal

Serves 2

This is a really delicious and easy to prepare fish dish. You could use fresh tiger prawns or scallops in this recipe, in which case you would need to add them to the pan along with the monkfish.

½ red pepper	1 bay leaf
1 medium courgette	400g tin chopped tomatoes
1 garlic clove	225g/8oz monkfish
1 tbsp olive oil	1 tbsp chopped fresh parsley
½ tsp dried oregano	6 cherry tomatoes
½ tsp dried basil	85g/3oz cooked prawns
½ tsp fennel seeds	salt and pepper

1   Slice the pepper and courgette and press the garlic clove. Sweat these in the olive oil until the vegetables are partly cooked.
2   Add the oregano, basil, fennel seeds, bay leaf and the tinned tomatoes. Bring to the boil and simmer for 2 minutes.
3   Remove the skin from the fish and cut it into bite-sized pieces. Add the pieces to the pan along with the fresh parsley and simmer for approximately 5 minutes or until the monkfish is cooked.
4   Cut the cherry tomatoes in half and add to the pan along with the prawns. Bring to the boil but do not continue cooking. Remove the bay leaf and season to taste with salt and pepper. Serve with rice and a green salad.

cooking without made easy

Thai Monkfish with Green Rice
Serves 2

Ground almonds are used to thicken the coconut sauce in this recipe, but you can omit them if you wish. For a change from mushrooms, try other vegetables in this dish – for example, baby sweetcorn, sugar snap peas or sliced courgettes.

1 medium onion	30g/1oz ground almonds (optional)
1 tbsp olive oil	salt and pepper
225g/8oz button mushrooms	
2 tbsp Thai Green Curry Paste (see page 106)	GREEN RICE:
	170g/6oz uncooked basmati rice
285g/10oz monkfish	1 bay leaf
1 level tsp Chinese five spice powder	1 tbsp chopped fresh coriander
1 tbsp chopped fresh coriander	1 tbsp chopped fresh mint
240ml/8fl oz coconut milk	

1 Dice the onion and sweat this in the olive oil until it begins to soften. Halve or quarter the mushrooms (if large) and add to the pan along with the curry paste. Sweat the ingredients for a few more minutes.
2 Meanwhile, boil the basmati rice with the bay leaf.
3 Remove any skin from the monkfish and cut the flesh into bite-sized pieces. Add the fish to the vegetables, along with the five spice powder, coriander and coconut milk.
4 Bring to the boil and simmer for approximately 5 minutes or until the monkfish is just cooked. Add the ground almonds, if using, to thicken the sauce. Season to taste with salt and pepper.
5 Drain the basmati rice, remove the bay leaf and mix in the coriander and mint. Serve the fish with the green rice.

Pasta with Smoked Salmon and Vegetables

Serves 2

This dish lends itself to substitutions. Other pastas or milk could be used and other vegetables, such as sweetcorn, broad beans and courgettes. You could add some cooked prawns instead of, or as well as, the salmon. It's a good idea to toss the pasta in a little olive oil if it is ready before you have cooked the other ingredients, as this prevents it sticking together. If you are using wheat pasta you won't need as much – 170g/6oz will provide two good-sized portions.

225g/8oz rice pasta	1 rounded tbsp corn or rice flour
1 small onion	425ml/15fl oz soya milk
1 red pepper	115g/4oz smoked salmon
1 tbsp olive oil	1 tbsp tamari or fish sauce (optional)
55g/2oz mushrooms	salt and pepper
115g/4oz mangetout	parsley to garnish

1   Cook the pasta according to the manufacturer's instructions.
2   Dice the onion and slice the pepper and sweat these in the olive oil until they begin to soften. Cut the mushrooms into halves or quarters if large and add to the pan along with the mangetout. Continue to sweat until all the vegetables are almost cooked.
3   Combine the flour and soya milk and add to the pan. Bring to the boil, stirring continuously, then turn the heat to low.
4   Cut the smoked salmon into small pieces and add to the sauce along with the tamari or fish sauce and the pasta.
5   Season to taste (you won't need salt if using tamari or fish sauce) and serve in pasta bowls, garnished with the parsley.

Herb- and Nut-Crusted Tuna
Serves 2

This recipe is extremely simple to make. Tuna and nuts make a good combination and the coriander gives the tuna extra piquancy. It's stylish enough to serve to special guests but only takes minutes to cook.

2 tbsp chopped almonds	2 x 140g/5oz tuna steaks
2 tbsp chopped fresh coriander	1 tbsp olive oil
salt and pepper	

1 Set the oven temperature to 200°C/400°F/Gas Mark 6.
2 Mix the almonds, coriander and a sprinkle of salt and pepper on a plate.
3 Dry the tuna steaks on kitchen paper and brush both sides with olive oil. Dip each side of the steaks in the nuts and herbs to coat.
4 Place the steaks on a baking tray and bake at the top of the oven, uncovered, for approximately 10 minutes. The time required will depend on the thickness of the steaks. Tuna fish should still be slightly pink inside when served – do not over-cook the steaks or they will become tough.
5 Serve immediately with salad or vegetables.

Vegetarian Main Courses

Spaghetti with Mushrooms, Spinach and Cherry Tomatoes

Serves 2

This is a really quick and easy dish to prepare. If you use dried, as opposed to bottled, sun-dried tomatoes, soften them in a little boiling water. You could add olives instead of, or as well as, the sun-dried tomatoes. Pasta is available in lots of alternatives to wheat, such as buckwheat, rice and corn. If you do use wheat pasta, you won't need quite as much – try 170g/6oz.

1 garlic clove	2 tbsp good quality olive oil
115g/4oz mushrooms	115g/4oz baby spinach leaves
115g/4oz cherry tomatoes	handful basil leaves
4 sun-dried tomatoes	salt and pepper
225g/8oz wheat-free spaghetti	2 tbsp toasted pine nuts

1 Press the garlic clove, slice the mushrooms, halve the cherry tomatoes and finely dice the sun-dried tomatoes.
2 Cook the spaghetti according to the directions, then drain and toss in 1 tablespoon of olive oil to prevent it from sticking.
3 Sweat the garlic, mushrooms and spinach in the remaining tablespoon of olive oil until the vegetables are just cooked.
4 Add the cherry tomatoes, sun-dried tomatoes and spaghetti. Tear the basil leaves into small pieces and add these.
5 Stir gently to combine and season to taste with salt and pepper. Place in pasta bowls, garnish with the pine nuts and serve.

Vegetable Moussaka
Serves 2

This dish is far easier to prepare than it first looks, and it can be prepared ahead of time and kept in the fridge until you are ready. If you want to use dried lentils, use 115g/4oz and cook in 570ml/1 pint of stock until soft and just starting to break up. When cooked, there should be 425ml/15fl oz of lentils and their juices, so add a little water if too much evaporates. If cheese is acceptable, grate a little on the surface before the final bake.

1 onion	400g tin chopped tomatoes
1 garlic clove	2 tbsp tomato purée (optional)
2 tbsp olive oil	1 small aubergine
115g/4oz mushrooms or 1 red pepper	1 egg
½ tsp dried rosemary or 1 tsp fresh	140g/5fl oz soya or other yogurt
½ tsp dried thyme or 1 tsp fresh	60ml/2fl oz soya or other milk
400g tin green or brown lentils	salt and pepper
	chopped parsley to garnish

1   Set the oven temperature to 200°C/400°F/Gas Mark 6.
2   Finely dice the onion and press the garlic clove and sweat these in 1 table-spoon of olive oil until they begin to soften.
3   Finely dice the mushrooms or pepper and add to the pan. Continue to sweat for another 5 minutes.
4   Add the rosemary, thyme, lentils (and their juices), tinned tomatoes and tomato purée and stir to combine.
5   Cut the aubergine into 5mm/¼in slices. Cover the base of a deep-sided lasagne dish with half of the lentil mixture and then half of the aubergine slices. Repeat the process, finishing with a second layer of aubergine.
6   Brush the aubergine with the remaining olive oil and cover the dish with foil. Bake for approximately 1 hour or until the aubergine slices are cooked, then remove the foil.
7   Beat the egg and combine with the yogurt and milk. Season with salt and pepper and pour over the aubergine. The moussaka mixture may still be visible in places, but that's fine. Bake for a further 15–20 minutes or until the topping is set.
8   Garnish with parsley and serve.

Vegetable Lasagne

Serves 2

Various types of wheat-free, lasagne-style pastas are now available. Substitute one of these for the aubergine used in the previous recipe. Follow the previous recipe making the changes listed below.

1   Place a third of the vegetable and lentil mixture into a lasagne dish, then add a layer of pasta. Repeat this process and then finish with the final third of the vegetable and lentil mixture.
2   Cover the lasagne with foil and bake for approximately 30–40 minutes. This will depend on how long your chosen pasta takes to cook. Remove the foil, add the topping and bake for a further 15 minutes or until the topping is set.

Roasted Stuffed Peppers
Serves 2

This dish is quick and easy to prepare and, if you line the baking tin with foil, there's very little washing up! Try substituting fresh fennel for the onions to produce another wholesome dish.

2 large red peppers	⅛ tsp chilli powder
2 medium onions	1 tsp dried oregano or 1 tbsp fresh
2 garlic cloves	2 tbsp chopped fresh coriander
400g tin chopped tomatoes	salt and black pepper
1 tsp paprika	fresh coriander to garnish

1 Set the oven temperature to 200°C/400°F/Gas Mark 6.
2 Cut the peppers in half lengthwise, cutting through the stalks and leaving these in place. Deseed the peppers and peel and cut the onions into quarters.
3 Press the garlic cloves and mix with the tomatoes, paprika, chilli powder, oregano and coriander. Season with salt and pepper.
4 Place the peppers in a shallow ovenproof dish, cut side uppermost. Place a tablespoon of the tomato mixture in each pepper, then two quarters of an onion on top.
5 Pour the rest of the tomato mixture over and around the peppers. Cover with foil and bake for approximately 1 hour or until the onions and peppers have softened.
6 Garnish the peppers with coriander and serve with salad, rice or potatoes.

Mexican Tacos with Avocado and Tomato Salsa

Serves 2

For convenience, you can use tinned beans in this recipe, though freshly cooked ones do taste better. I often cook a large batch of beans and then freeze them for future use. To make these tacos really special, serve them topped with the sour cream from page 148 or, for those who can tolerate dairy produce, with grated cheese.

1 medium onion	salt and pepper
½–1 red chilli	2 large tomatoes
1 large garlic clove	1 avocado
1 tbsp olive oil	1 tbsp lemon juice
285g/10oz cooked black eye beans or 400g tin of beans, washed and drained	6 taco shells

1 Finely dice the onion and chilli and press the garlic clove. Sweat these in the olive oil until they are cooked.
2 Add the beans and stir while they heat through. Mash a few of the beans so that they break up and the mixture starts to stick together. Season the beans to taste with salt and pepper.
3 Finely dice the tomatoes (you can skin them if you prefer). Finely dice the avocado flesh and toss this in the lemon juice to prevent it browning. Combine the avocado with the tomatoes and season to taste with salt and pepper.
4 Heat the taco shells, according to the instructions on the packet, until crisp.
5 Divide the beans between the taco shells then pile the avocado mixture on top. Serve immediately with salad.

Creamy Vegetable
and Cashew Nut Risotto

Serves 2

It normally takes an age to make a risotto, as the liquid is added gradually to uncooked risotto rice. This is the cheat's version, which I often make when I have some ready-cooked rice. Short grain rice produces a creamier risotto but long grain is quite acceptable.

115g/4oz whole cashew nuts	½ tsp dried thyme or 1 tsp fresh
2 medium carrots	½ tsp dried marjoram or 1 tsp fresh
1 medium onion	140ml/5fl oz coconut milk
1 garlic clove	140ml/5fl oz water
1 tbsp olive oil	400g/14oz cooked brown rice
55g/2oz button mushrooms or	(200g/7oz uncooked)
115g/4oz courgette	salt and pepper
55g/2oz fresh or frozen peas	2 tbsp chopped fresh parsley

1 Toast the cashews in the oven or under a hot grill until golden brown. Watch carefully as they quickly burn.
2 Finely dice the carrots and onion and press the garlic clove. Sweat these in the olive oil until they begin to soften.
3 Dice the mushrooms or courgette and add to the pan along with the peas and herbs. Continue to sweat until the vegetables are almost cooked.
4 Add the coconut milk, water and rice. Bring to the boil and simmer until you have a creamy textured risotto with some residual juices. This will take 5–10 minutes.
5 Season the risotto to taste with salt and pepper and mix in the nuts and most of the parsley. Garnish the risotto with the remaining parsley and serve.

Speedy Asparagus, Pea and Pine Nut Risotto
Serves 2

This recipe makes a delightful supper dish in the summer, when fresh asparagus is in season. When asparagus isn't available, substitute 225g/8oz green beans. If acceptable, toss a good knob of butter in the risotto before serving and sprinkle with Parmesan flakes, or add 1 table-spoon of tamari sauce.

30g/1oz pine nuts	240ml/8fl oz good quality stock
1 medium onion	455g/1lb cooked rice (225g/8oz
1 garlic clove	uncooked)
1 tbsp olive oil	1 tbsp chopped fresh parsley
1 bunch asparagus	salt and pepper
225g/8oz fresh or frozen peas	lemon wedges to garnish

1 Toast the pine nuts in the oven or under a hot grill until golden brown.
2 Finely dice the onion and press the garlic clove and sweat these in the olive oil until the onion begins to soften.
3 Cut the bottoms off the asparagus stalks then cut into 2.5cm/1in lengths. Add to the pan along with the peas and continue to sweat for a few minutes. Add the stock and simmer until the vegetables are almost cooked.
4 Add the rice and parsley and bring to the boil. Simmer for approximately 5 minutes or until the stock is absorbed and the vegetables are cooked.
5 Season the risotto to taste with salt and pepper and serve in bowls, garnished with the pine nuts and lemon wedges.

Speedy Spinach and Pumpkin Risotto
Serves 2

This is a tasty and substantial risotto to serve at the end of summer, when the nights start to draw in and you need some warm, comforting food. It's even more delicious sprinkled with Parmesan flakes, if these are acceptable. Butternut squash can be substituted for the pumpkin when this is not in season.

1 onion	1 tsp grated lemon rind (optional)
1 garlic clove	140ml/5fl oz good quality stock
1 tbsp olive oil	400g/14oz cooked brown rice
455g/1lb pumpkin flesh	(200g/7oz uncooked)
115g/4oz baby spinach leaves	1 tbsp chopped fresh parsley
1 tbsp chopped fresh oregano or 1 tsp	salt and pepper
dried oregano	parsley to garnish

1   Dice the onion and press the garlic clove. Sweat these in the olive oil until the onion begins to soften.
2   Deseed the pumpkin and cut the flesh into 2.5cm/1in cubes (you don't need to peel the pumpkin unless the skin is marked or tough). Add to the onion and continue to sweat the vegetables, stirring occasionally, until the pumpkin is just cooked. This takes a little while so don't turn the heat up too high and try to rush it.
3   Add the spinach, oregano, lemon rind and the stock. Bring to the boil and simmer until the spinach is cooked and the pumpkin is starting to break up.
4   Add the rice and parsley and heat through. Season to taste with salt and pepper and serve in individual bowls, garnished with parsley.

Spicy Thai Vegetables
with Rice Noodles
Serves 2

This recipe is another favourite of mine – it's a wonderful combination of colours, textures and flavours. Non-vegetarians could add chicken, prawns or egg (in the form of a diced omelette) and ½ tablespoon of fish sauce as well as, or instead of, the tamari sauce.

225g/8oz ribbon rice noodles	1 tbsp tamari sauce (optional)
2 tbsp olive oil	2 tbsp lemon juice
2 garlic cloves	140ml/¼ pint stock or water
2.5cm/1in piece ginger	1 tbsp chopped fresh parsley
2 medium leeks	2 tbsp chopped fresh basil or coriander
1 red pepper	2 handfuls beansprouts
115g/4oz button mushrooms (optional)	55g/2oz roasted salted peanuts
1 red chilli	parsley or coriander to garnish
1 carrot	

1 Soak the noodles for 20 minutes in warm water then drain and toss in 1 tablespoon of olive oil to prevent them sticking together.
2 Press the garlic cloves; grate the ginger; slice the leeks, red pepper and mushrooms; finely dice the chilli and cut the carrot into slivers using a potato peeler.
3 Sweat these in the remaining tablespoon of olive oil, adding the mushrooms last of all, until they are all just cooked.
4 Add the noodles, tamari, lemon juice, stock or water and fresh herbs. Bring to the boil and heat through.
5 Pile into individual serving bowls and scatter the beansprouts and peanuts over the top. Garnish with herbs and serve.

Tofu Noodle Hot-Pot
Serves 2

This truly scrumptious mix of ingredients is enhanced by a fragrant stock. Eat it with a spoon and fork and, if acceptable, use some crusty bread to mop up the juices. Lots of other vegetables can be used in this dish, such as spinach, beansprouts, mangetout, mushrooms, water chestnuts and broad beans.

115g/4oz ribbon rice noodles	850ml/1½ pints vegetable stock
2 tbsp olive oil	285ml/½ pint coconut milk
1 garlic clove	85g/3oz peas, fresh or frozen
1 bunch spring onions	115g/4oz baby sweetcorn
1 red pepper	125g/4½oz plain tofu
2.5cm/1in piece ginger	2 tbsp chopped fresh basil
½–1 red chilli	1 tbsp chopped fresh coriander plus
2 tbsp smooth peanut butter (or other	extra to garnish
nut butter)	salt and pepper
1 tbsp tamari sauce (optional)	55g/2oz toasted cashew nuts
1 tsp grated lemon rind	

1 Soak the rice noodles in warm water for 20 minutes. Drain and toss in 1 tablespoon of olive oil to prevent them from sticking.
2 Press the garlic clove, slice the spring onions and red pepper, grate the ginger and very finely dice the red chilli. Sweat these in 1 tablespoon of olive oil until they begin to soften.
3 Add the peanut butter, tamari, lemon rind, vegetable stock, coconut milk, peas and sweetcorn. Dice the tofu and add to the pan along with the basil and coriander. Bring to the boil and simmer for 5 minutes.
4 Add the rice noodles, heat through and season to taste with salt and pepper.
5 Serve in individual pasta bowls, garnished with the cashews and coriander.

Tofu, Pineapple and Cashew Nut Stir-Fry

Serves 2

This colourful and unusual stir-fry can be served over rice or millet, or tossed with rice noodles. Use tinned pineapple chunks in fruit juice. If there is insufficient pineapple juice from the tin, squeeze a few pineapple chunks to produce more.

85g/3oz whole cashew nuts	115g/4oz pineapple chunks
250g/9oz plain tofu	salt and pepper
½ red pepper	parsley to garnish
1 courgette	
85g/3oz button mushrooms or	MARINADE:
85g/3oz mangetout	1 garlic clove, pressed
4 spring onions	2.5cm/1in piece ginger, grated
1 medium carrot	1 tbsp olive oil
1 tbsp olive oil	1 tsp sesame oil
140ml/5fl oz pineapple juice	salt and pepper
1 tsp corn or rice flour	

1   Toast the cashew nuts in the oven or under a hot grill until golden brown.
2   Cube the tofu and press with kitchen paper to remove the excess mois-
    ture. Mix together the marinade ingredients and toss with the tofu. Leave
    to marinate as long as possible but at least while you prepare the other
    ingredients.
3   Cut the red pepper and courgette into strips, half or quarter the mush-
    rooms, slice the spring onions and cut the carrot into slivers using a potato
    peeler.
4   Sweat the vegetables and tofu in the olive oil, starting with the pepper,
    courgette and carrot and adding the mushrooms, spring onions and tofu
    partway through cooking.
5   Mix the pineapple juice and flour together and add to the stir-fry along with
    the pineapple chunks. Bring to the boil and simmer until all the vegetables
    are cooked.
6   Season to taste with salt and pepper and serve in individual bowls,
    garnished with parsley and cashew nuts.

Spaghetti with Gingered Vegetables and Cashews

Serves 2

Spaghetti made from wheat-free ingredients, such as buckwheat and corn, is now widely available. If you are not vegetarian, try adding ½ tablespoon fish sauce to the spaghetti once it's cooked – this gives it a really good flavour. You can serve the vegetables and nuts with rice instead of spaghetti if you prefer.

55g/2oz whole cashew nuts	170g/6oz spaghetti
680g/1½lb selection of vegetables	½ tsp sesame oil
e.g. broccoli, mushrooms, onion,	2 tbsp good quality olive oil
spring onion, peppers, courgettes,	2 tbsp chopped fresh basil or
peas, mangetout, broad beans,	coriander
celery, baby sweetcorn, spinach	½ tbsp tamari sauce (optional)
2.5cm/1in piece ginger	½ tbsp lemon juice
1 garlic clove	salt and pepper

1 Toast the cashews in the oven or under a hot grill until they are golden brown.
2 Cut all the vegetables into small pieces that will cook in approximately the same amount of time. Grate the ginger and press the garlic clove.
3 Cook the spaghetti according to the packet instructions and drain. Toss the spaghetti with the sesame oil, 1 tablespoon of olive oil, the basil or coriander, tamari and lemon juice.
4 Sweat the garlic, ginger and vegetables in the remaining olive oil until they are soft and starting to brown.
5 Mix the vegetables and spaghetti and season to taste with salt and pepper. Serve in individual bowls, garnished with the cashew nuts.

Baked Potatoes with Humous and Roasted Vegetables

Serves 2

I love baked potatoes and find them a really useful convenience food. In summer, when baby new potatoes are all you can find, look out for Cyprus potatoes – they are always larger. Do allow extra time when baking new potatoes, as they do always seem to take longer than old ones. The recipe for humous will make lots so you will have some left over for the next day or to freeze. Halve the quantities if you don't want to make extra. Humous is readily available in supermarkets and the ingredients are usually quite acceptable, so cheat by all means.

2 large baking potatoes	HUMOUS:
900g/2lb selection of vegetables e.g.	400g tin chickpeas, drained
butternut squash, onions, courgettes,	2 tbsp lemon juice
peppers, carrots, aubergine, sweet	3 tbsp tahini
potato, fennel	1 garlic clove, pressed
2 tbsp olive oil	approx. 60ml/2fl oz water
	salt and pepper

1   Prick the potatoes with a fork and bake at 200°C/400°F/Gas Mark 6 for approximately 60 minutes or until soft when pressed.
2   Cut the vegetables into pieces that will all cook in a similar time and toss these in the olive oil. Place on a baking tray and bake, along with the potatoes, for approximately 40 minutes.
3   To make the humous, process the chickpeas, lemon juice, tahini and garlic until smooth and creamy. Add sufficient water to give the humous a soft dropping consistency and season to taste with salt and pepper.
4   Cut the potatoes in half and mash the flesh a little with a fork. Pile the humous onto the potatoes then pile the roasted vegetables on top and around. Serve immediately, with salad if desired.

Baked Potatoes with Sour Cream and Roasted Vegetables

Follow the previous recipe for the potatoes and vegetables, substituting the Sour Cream recipe below for the humous. The Butterbean and Thyme Pâté from the starters section can also be used in this recipe (though you'll need to add a few tablespoons of water to make the pâté a little softer).

SOUR CREAM:	⅛ tsp vanilla extract
175g/6oz firm silken tofu	⅛ tsp salt
1 tbsp lemon juice	2 tbsp soya milk

1   To make the sour cream, process or beat all the ingredients together until they are smooth and creamy.
2   Cut the baked potatoes in half and mash the flesh a little with a fork.
3   Pile the sour cream into the potatoes then pile the roasted vegetables on top. Serve immediately, with salad if desired.

Baked Potatoes with Sour Cream and Garlic Mushrooms

Serves 2

Garlic mushrooms are delicious served with sour cream.

2 large baking potatoes	1 large garlic clove
Sour Cream (see page 148)	1 tsp olive oil
285g/10oz mushrooms (preferably	1 tsp butter or margarine
field)	salt and pepper

1 Prick the potatoes with a fork and bake at 200°C/400°F/Gas Mark 6 for approximately 60 minutes or until soft when pressed.
2 Make the sour cream according to the recipe.
3 Cut the mushrooms into even-sized pieces and press the garlic clove. Sweat the mushrooms and garlic in the olive oil and butter or margarine until the mushrooms begin to soften and the juices just start to run.
4 Season the mushrooms to taste with salt and pepper.
5 Cut the potatoes in half and mash the flesh a little with a fork. Pile the sour cream into the potatoes and top with the garlic mushrooms. Serve at once with salad.

Baked Potatoes with Roasted Onions and Pesto Dressing

Quarter 4 onions and toss in 1 tablespoon of olive oil. Roast on a baking tray at 200°C/400°F/Gas Mark 6 for approximately 30 minutes or until soft and starting to brown. Serve with baked potatoes and the Pesto Dressing from page 82 of the salad section or a proprietary pesto dressing, if this is acceptable.

Tahini-Baked Sweet Potatoes with Roasted Vegetables

Serves 2

In this recipe, the cooked sweet potato flesh is mixed with tahini and piled back into the skins to produce a really delicious combination of flavours and a wonderfully creamy texture. This is comfort food with attitude, according to a friend of mine. Mushrooms and tomatoes can be added to the roasted vegetables, but add them partway through cooking as they don't take long to bake.

2 large sweet potatoes	2 tbsp olive oil
900g/2lb selection of vegetables	2 tbsp tahini
e.g. courgettes, peppers, onions,	salt and pepper
aubergine, fennel, celery	2 tbsp toasted pine nuts

1 Prick the sweet potatoes with a fork and bake whole at 200°C/400°F/Gas Mark 6 for approximately 1 hour or until soft when pressed. The length of time will depend on the size of potatoes.

2 Cut the vegetables into chunks that will cook in a similar amount of time. Toss these in the olive oil to coat and then place the vegetables on a baking tray. Bake in the oven, along with the potatoes, for approximately 40 minutes or until the vegetables are just cooked.

3 Cut the baked potatoes in half and scoop out most of the centres into a bowl. Add the tahini and mash the mixture until creamy. Season the mixture to taste with salt and pepper and pile it back into the potato shells.

4 Garnish the baked potatoes with pine nuts and serve with the roasted vegetables.

Egg and Chips
Serves 2

My husband used to ask for egg and chips as his birthday treat in the days when I refused to have a chip pan in the house. Since I discovered this healthy way of producing chips we have them more often – with eggs, nature's best convenience food. I like to serve egg and chips with the ratatouille from page 157. They go surprisingly well together.

3 large potatoes	4 eggs
1 tbsp olive oil	

1   Heat the oven to 200°C/400°F/Gas Mark 6.
2   Peel and chip the potatoes and dry on a clean tea towel or kitchen paper. Place in a bowl with the olive oil and toss to coat. Place the chips in lines on one or two baking trays, with a small gap between each chip. Bake in the oven for approximately 30–40 minutes until the chips are golden brown and soft when pressed. The length of time does vary with the type of potato.
3   Cook the eggs in your favourite way. I prefer fried eggs with chips but I use a non-stick pan so I only need 1 teaspoon of oil.
4   Serve the egg and chips hot.

Omelette and Chips
Serves 2

For an up-market version of egg and chips try one of the following omelettes. It's such a quick and easy meal and delicious served with a green salad or the ratatouille on page 157.

3 large potatoes	salt and pepper
4 eggs	2 tsp olive oil
2 tbsp water	

1 Make the chips as directed in the Egg and Chips recipe (page 151).
2 Whisk the eggs with the water and salt and pepper.
3 Heat 1 teaspoon of oil in an omelette pan and add half of the egg mixture. Cook over a medium high heat until the base of the omelette starts to cook. Then, using a spatula, push the cooked egg towards the middle of the pan allowing the still-soft egg to run to the base. Continue with this process until the omelette is only just set and starting to brown on the base. Fold in half, turn out onto a warm plate and serve with the chips. Make the second omelette in the same way.

Tomato and Chive Omelette

Add a sliced tomato and a teaspoon of chopped chives to each omelette halfway through cooking and proceed as above.

Spring Onion, Olive
and Sun-Dried Tomato Omelette

Add 1 finely chopped spring onion, 3 finely chopped olives and 1 chopped sun-dried tomato to each omelette partway through cooking and proceed as above.

Mushroom Omelette

Soften 115g/4oz mushrooms in a little olive oil, butter or margarine and season with a little salt and pepper. Add half to each omelette partway through cooking and proceed as above.

Herb Omelette

Add a heaped tablespoon of chopped fresh herbs to each omelette part-way through cooking and proceed as above. Choose from parsley, chives, basil, tarragon, fennel, dill or a mixture of these.

Baby Spinach, Pea
and Broad Bean Omelette

Sweat a handful of baby spinach leaves, 3 tablespoons of peas and 3 tablespoons of broad beans in a teaspoon of olive oil until they are just cooked. Add half of the mixture to each omelette partway through cooking and proceed as above.

This is delicious made with fresh peas and broad beans when they are in season but frozen vegetables are quite acceptable. If using frozen peas and beans, add them to the pan with the spinach and they will defrost while the spinach cooks.

All-In-One Courgette and Mushroom Quiche

Serves 4

This pastry-less quiche is quick and easy to make, yet truly scrumptious. The recipe serves four as it's not easy to find a small, deep quiche dish and the quiche freezes well anyway. For those who feel a quiche needs cheese, 85g/3oz of grated cheese can be added, though it really isn't necessary as the quiche is so good.

1 onion	5 eggs
1 garlic clove	115g/4oz gluten-free flour (or rice
1 tbsp olive oil	flour)
115g/4oz mushrooms	1 rounded tsp baking powder
115g/4oz butter or margarine	2 tbsp chopped fresh parsley
3 medium courgettes	salt and pepper

1 Grease a 25cm/10in, deep flan dish and set the oven temperature to 170°C/325°F/Gas Mark 3.
2 Dice the onion and press the garlic clove and sweat these in the olive oil until the onion begins to soften and brown.
3 Slice the mushrooms, add to the pan and continue to sweat until the mushrooms begin to soften.
4 Cut the butter or margarine into small pieces, add to the pan and leave on a low heat until the butter has melted.
5 Grate the courgettes on a large-holed grater.
6 Beat or process the eggs, flour and baking powder together.
7 Combine all the ingredients and season with salt and pepper.
8 Pour into the flan dish and bake for 35–40 minutes or until the quiche is just set and golden brown. Serve warm or cold with salad.

All-in-One Leek and Sweetcorn Quiche
Serves 4

If you wish to make a smaller quiche, halve the quantities and reduce the cooking time. This quiche does, however, keep well for a second day's serving and also freezes beautifully. You can add 85g/3oz of grated cheese if this is acceptable, but it really isn't necessary as the quiche is so tasty.

1 medium onion	5 eggs
1 garlic clove	115g/4oz gluten-free flour (or rice
340g/12oz leeks (mainly white stems)	flour)
1 tbsp olive oil	1 rounded tsp baking powder
225g/8oz sweetcorn	2 tbsp chopped fresh parsley
115g/4oz butter or margarine	salt and pepper

1   Grease a 25cm/10in, deep flan dish and set the oven temperature to 170°C/325°F/Gas Mark 3.
2   Dice the onion, press the garlic clove and slice the leeks into 1cm/½in slices. Sweat the vegetables in the olive oil until they begin to soften.
3   Add the sweetcorn. Cut the butter or margarine into small pieces and add this to the pan, too. Leave on a low heat until the butter has melted.
4   Beat or process the eggs, flour and baking powder together.
5   Combine all the ingredients and season with salt and pepper.
6   Pour into the flan dish and bake for 35–40 minutes or until the quiche is just set and starting to turn golden brown. Serve warm or cold with salad.

Ratatouille with Passata and Cherry Tomatoes

Serves 3–4

This recipe makes a substantial amount of ratatouille but to lessen it means using part of a container of passata, which seems such a waste. Half the quantities if you like. Add 115g/4oz of beans (butterbeans, chickpeas, cannellini) to make this ratatouille a more balanced main course. I make lots of ratatouille at the end of summer, when the ingredients needed are cheap and plentiful, and I always freeze some to use mid-winter.

2 large onions	500ml/17½fl oz passata (sieved
2 garlic cloves	tomatoes)
1 tbsp olive oil	225g/8oz cherry tomatoes
4 medium courgettes	salt and pepper
1 red and 1 yellow pepper	

1   Cut the onions into large chunks and press the garlic cloves. Sweat these in the olive oil until they begin to soften.
2   Slice the courgettes and peppers and add these to the pan. Continue to sweat the vegetables until they are all beginning to soften.
3   Add the passata, bring to the boil and simmer until all the vegetables are just cooked. Add the cherry tomatoes and heat through. The ratatouille is ready when some of the cherry tomatoes are starting to burst and some are still whole. Season to taste with salt and pepper.
4   Serve with rice or pasta or as a vegetable accompaniment to other meals.

Spicy Vegetable Gumbo
Serves 2

If you are vegetarian or vegan and want to increase the protein content of this recipe, add 115g/4oz tofu before cooking. If you cannot tolerate tomatoes, substitute a tin of green lentils, including the juices. Cajun spice contains paprika, basil, fennel, cumin, mustard and cayenne and gives a lovely flavour to this dish. If you prefer your gumbo hotter, add more Cajun seasoning. Okra is available from supermarkets and oriental grocers.

1 medium onion	1 garlic clove
2 sticks celery	1 rounded tsp Cajun seasoning
1 red pepper	400g tin chopped tomatoes
1 fresh or frozen corn cob	425ml/¾ pint vegetable stock
1 large carrot	½ tbsp tamari sauce (optional)
115g/4oz okra	2 tbsp chopped fresh parsley

1 Set the oven temperature to 200°C/400°F/Gas Mark 6.
2 Cut the onion, celery, pepper, corn cob and carrot into bite-sized chunks, top and tail the okra and press the garlic clove. Place the vegetables in a casserole dish.
3 Mix the Cajun seasoning with the tomatoes, stock and tamari sauce (if using). Add to the casserole and mix to combine.
4 Cover the casserole and cook for approximately 1 hour or until the vegetables are just cooked.
5 Mix in the parsley and serve with rice, millet or baked potatoes.

Vegetable Goulash
Serves 2

This is a classic vegetable stew, bursting with wonderful colours and flavours. If you wish, you can sweat the vegetables in 1 tablespoon of olive oil before adding the rest of the ingredients. Add 115g/4oz of beans (kidney, butterbeans or chickpeas) for extra protein if you are vegetarian or vegan.

1 onion	400g tin chopped tomatoes
1 garlic clove	1 dsp smoked paprika
225g/½lb new potatoes	1 bay leaf
565g/1¼lb selection of vegetables	salt and pepper
e.g. peppers, courgettes, cauliflower,	140g/5oz soya yogurt
carrots, parsnips, celery, mushrooms,	1 tbsp chopped fresh parsley
sweetcorn, broccoli, butternut squash	

1 Set the oven temperature to 200°C/400°F/Gas Mark 6.
2 Cut the onion into large chunks, press the garlic clove and halve or quarter the new potatoes.
3 Cut the selection of vegetables into largish chunks that will cook in roughly the same amount of time. Place all the vegetables in a casserole dish.
4 Mix the tomatoes with the smoked paprika and add to the casserole with the bay leaf. Mix to combine.
5 Cover the casserole and cook for approximately 50–60 minutes or until the vegetables are just tender. Add a little water near the end of cooking if the mixture seems a little dry.
6 Place in individual dishes, stir in a swirl of yogurt, sprinkle with parsley and serve.

Mushroom and Butterbean Stroganoff
Serves 2

If you use tinned butterbeans this really is a speedy meal. Other beans, or tofu, could be used instead of the butterbeans for a variation on this stroganoff.

1 onion	¼ tsp dried thyme
1 garlic clove	¼ tsp dried rosemary
1 tbsp olive oil	1 level tsp mustard
250g/9oz selection of mushrooms	225g/8oz soya yogurt
e.g. chestnut, shiitake, field	170g/6oz cooked butterbeans
¼ tsp grated nutmeg	1 tbsp chopped fresh parsley
½ tsp dried basil	salt and pepper

1 Cut the onions into chunks and press the garlic clove. Sweat these in the olive oil until the onions are soft and beginning to brown.
2 Cut the mushrooms into halves or quarters depending on their size.
3 Add these to the pan along with the nutmeg, basil, thyme and rosemary. Continue to cook until the mushrooms are just starting to soften.
4 Combine the yogurt and the mustard and add to the pan along with the butterbeans. Heat through gently but do not over-cook or the yogurt may begin to separate.
5 Add the parsley and season to taste with salt and pepper. Serve with rice, quinoa or millet.

Creamy Tahini and Vegetable Casserole
Serves 2

Rich, creamy and wholesome, this dish is just right for a cold winter's evening. Other vegetables that could be used include fennel, leeks, parsnips, mushrooms and butternut squash. Why not put some potatoes into the oven to bake along with the casserole then you can have some time off while the meal is cooking?

1 onion	3 rounded tbsp tahini
3 sticks celery	425ml/¾ pint vegetable stock
1 garlic clove	400g tin blackeye beans
1 tbsp olive oil	salt and pepper
1 large carrot	1 tbsp chopped fresh parsley
¼ celeriac	extra parsley to garnish
1 red pepper	

1   Set the oven temperature to 200°C/400°F/Gas Mark 6.
2   Cut the onion and celery into chunks and press the garlic clove.
3   Sweat the onions, celery and garlic in the olive oil in a casserole dish until the vegetables begin to soften.
4   Cut the carrot, celeriac and pepper into bite-sized chunks and add to the casserole. Dissolve the tahini in the vegetable stock and add this, too.
5   Add half the blackeye beans to the casserole and mash the remaining beans with your hands to break up before adding.
6   Add the tablespoon of parsley, cover the casserole and bake for 1 hour or until the vegetables are cooked. Don't worry if the mixture looks a little curdled when you remove it from the oven – it will become creamy once stirred.
7   Season to taste with salt and pepper (you won't need salt if you have used a stock cube) and serve garnished with parsley.

Butterbean and Vegetable Medley
Serves 2

This is really speedy but tasty food – a sort of casserole cooked in a pan. Other vegetables that can be used in this dish include fennel, peppers and celery and you can use your favourite type of bean instead of the butterbeans.

1 onion	3 sun-dried tomatoes
handful French beans	400g tin butterbeans
1 large courgette	85ml/3fl oz stock or water
1 large carrot	1 tbsp chopped fresh herbs or 1 tsp
piece of broccoli	dried mixed herbs (e.g. basil, thyme,
1 garlic clove	rosemary, tarragon)
1 tbsp olive oil	salt and pepper
3 large tomatoes	

1 Cut the vegetables into pieces that will cook in a similar amount of time. Press the garlic clove.
2 Sweat the vegetables and garlic in the olive oil until they are starting to soften.
3 Dice the fresh tomatoes and the sun-dried tomatoes and add these to the pan along with the butterbeans, stock and herbs.
4 Bring to the boil, cover and simmer for 10–15 minutes or until the vegetables are tender. Season to taste with salt and pepper and serve in bowls.

Spiced Parsnips with Cashew Nuts
Serves 2

This very tasty winter evening dish is warm and filling. The first six ingredients are made into a paste that forms part of the sauce. If you don't have a processor, finely grate or chop the first five ingredients and use ground almonds instead of the cashew pieces.

2 garlic cloves	½ tsp cumin seeds
1 shallot	½ tsp ground coriander
2.5cm/1in piece ginger	½ tsp turmeric
½–1 green chilli	½ tsp garam masala
3 tbsp water	455g/1lb parsnips
30g/1oz cashew nuts pieces	425ml/¾ pint vegetable stock
1 medium onion	55g/2oz toasted whole cashew nuts
1 tbsp olive oil	2 tbsp chopped fresh coriander

1 Process the garlic, shallot, ginger, chilli, water and cashew nut pieces to form a paste.

2 Dice the onion and sweat this in the olive oil until it begins to soften. Add the spice paste, the cumin seeds, coriander, turmeric and garam masala and continue to cook for another few minutes, stirring frequently.

3 Cut three quarters of the parsnips into chunks and add to the pan along with the stock. Grate the remaining parsnips into the pan (this enables them to break down and form part of the sauce).

4 Bring the ingredients to the boil and simmer for approximately 20 minutes or until the parsnips are cooked and the sauce is thick.

5 Season to taste with salt and pepper then add the toasted cashew nuts (saving a few as a garnish) and fresh coriander.

6 Serve in individual bowls with rice and/or some soya yogurt and naan bread, if acceptable.

Thai Green Vegetable Curries

You can use ready-made Thai green curry paste in these recipes but I prefer to make my own (see page 106), as I prefer lots of flavour and not too much heat. It really is worth the effort to make this paste as the flavour is wonderful. If you use ready-made curry paste follow the manufacturer's instructions on the quantity to use. You can substitute soya yogurt or tinned tomatoes for the coconut milk in any of the following curries for a variation on the recipe. However, if you use soya yogurt, make sure that the vegetables are cooked before you add the yogurt as it will curdle if over-cooked. You will not need to use the ground almonds to thicken the curry if you use yogurt or tomatoes.

The variations on these curries are endless. Just use sufficient vegetables, beans or tofu in whatever combinations appeal to you and invent your own recipe.

Thai Cauliflower and Carrot Curry

Serves 2

2 medium carrots	285ml/10fl oz coconut milk
340g/¾lb cauliflower florets	30g/1oz ground almonds
1 tbsp olive oil	salt and pepper
3 heaped tbsp Thai Green Curry Paste	1 tbsp chopped fresh coriander
(see page 106)	

1 Cut the carrots into bite-sized pieces and sweat these and the cauliflower florets in the olive oil until they begin to soften.
2 Add the curry paste and sweat for a few more minutes.
3 Add the coconut milk, bring to the boil and simmer until the vegetables are just cooked.
4 Add the ground almonds to thicken the curry and season to taste with salt and pepper.
5 Garnish the curry with coriander and serve with rice, millet or quinoa.

Thai Mushroom and Courgette Curry

Substitute 455g/1lb sliced courgettes and 225g/½lb of halved or quartered mushrooms for the vegetables in the cauliflower and carrot curry then simply follow the recipe as before.

Thai Broccoli and Red Pepper Curry

Substitute 340g/12oz broccoli and 1 red pepper for the vegetables in the cauliflower and carrot curry and then follow the recipe as before.

Thai Butternut Squash and Spinach Curry

Serves 2

This curry follows the same principles as the other Thai curries but butternut squash is used to thicken the coconut milk instead of ground almonds. The spinach is added late in the recipe to prevent it from over-cooking.

565g/1¼lb butternut squash	285ml/10fl oz coconut milk
1 onion	115g/4oz baby spinach leaves
1 tbsp olive oil	2 tbsp chopped fresh coriander
3 heaped tbsp Thai Green Curry Paste	salt and pepper
(see page 106)	

1 Peel and deseed the butternut squash and cut it into bite-sized pieces.
2 Dice the onion and sweat this and the squash in the olive oil until the squash begins to soften. This takes a little while so don't turn the heat up too high and try to rush it.
3 Add the curry paste and sweat for a few more minutes.
4 Add the coconut milk, bring to the boil and simmer until the butternut squash is cooked. At this stage, mash a few pieces of the squash so that they break down to form part of the sauce.
5 Add the spinach leaves and the coriander and simmer for another few minutes until the spinach is just cooked. Do not continue to cook or the spinach will lose its bright green colour.
6 Season the curry to taste with salt and pepper and serve with rice, millet or quinoa.

Moroccan Vegetable Tagine
Serves 2

Vegetables combine wonderfully well with the sweet, sour and spicy flavours of Moroccan cooking. However, this dish will still be acceptable if you cannot tolerate the odd ingredient such as lemon or tomato purée. I love baked potatoes with this dish – as I can just pop them in the oven along with the tagine and have an hour off – but it goes equally well with rice or millet.

8 shallots	½ tsp ground cumin
½ red pepper	½ tsp ground coriander
2 sticks celery	½ tsp paprika
1 large carrot	½ tsp cinnamon
285g/10oz butternut squash	2 tbsp tomato purée (optional)
2.5cm/1in piece ginger	340ml/12fl oz vegetable stock
2 garlic cloves	1 tbsp chopped pickled lemon
8 dried apricots	salt and pepper
½ x 400g tin chickpeas	1 tbsp chopped fresh coriander

1 Set the oven temperature to 200°C/400°F/Gas Mark 6.
2 Peel the shallots, slice the red pepper and celery and cut the carrot into chunks. Place these in a casserole dish.
3 Peel and deseed the butternut squash and cut into bite-sized pieces. Cut one third of the pieces into tiny dice so that they will break down on cooking and form part of the sauce. Add all the squash to the casserole.
4 Grate the ginger and press the garlic cloves and add these to the casserole along with the dried apricots and rinsed chickpeas.
5 Mix the cumin, coriander, paprika, cinnamon and tomato purée with the stock and pour over the vegetables in the casserole dish.
6 Cover the casserole and cook for 50–60 minutes or until the vegetables are just cooked.
7 Stir in the pickled lemon and season to taste with salt and pepper. Garnish with the coriander and serve with rice, millet or baked potatoes.

Desserts

Pan-Fried Apples

Serves 2

I like to serve these apples warm with yogurt but they are equally good cold. As well as making a great dessert they're delicious served with porridge or muesli for breakfast.

> 3 dessert apples │ 1 tbsp walnuts to decorate
> 1 tbsp butter or margarine │

1 Wash the apples but do not peel them. Cut each apple into quarters and remove the core. Cut each apple quarter into thin slices.
2 Melt the butter or margarine in a frying pan and add the apples. Gently cook the apples for approximately 10 minutes or until they are golden brown and softened. Turn them once during cooking.
3 Serve the apples warm or cold, decorated with a few broken walnuts.

Strawberries in Red Grape Juice
Serves 2

When summer fruits are in season try making the following two easy-to-prepare desserts. The concentrated juice adds an intense fruity flavour while the fruit remains tangy but sweet.

400ml/14fl oz red grape juice | 400g/14oz strawberries

1 Place the grape juice in a pan, bring to the boil and simmer until it has reduced by half.
2 Halve or quarter the strawberries, depending on their size, and add to the grape juice when it has cooled a little but is still quite warm. The strawberries are meant to soften a little but not cook.
3 Allow the strawberries to cool and serve the strawberries and juice at room temperature or chilled if you prefer.

Nectarines and Cherries
in Red Grape Juice

Serves 2

400ml/14fl oz red grape juice	170g/6oz cherries
2 ripe nectarines	½ tsp vanilla extract

1 Place the grape juice in a pan, bring to the boil and simmer until it has reduced by half.
2 Stone and cut each nectarine into eight segments. Remove the stalks from the cherries.
3 Add the fruit and vanilla extract to the grape juice. Bring the fruit to the boil then immediately remove from the heat. Allow the mixture to cool in the pan. Serve at room temperature or chilled if you prefer.

Fresh Fruit Surprise
Serves 2

In this recipe, fresh fruit is hidden in a yogurt base, with ginger and toasted almonds providing a wonderful contrast of texture and flavour. Stem ginger is available bottled in syrup or crystallized. It does however contain a small amount of sugar so omit this if desired. You could add some dried fruit for an alternative to this recipe – try sultanas or cranberries, preferably soaked in boiling water until plump and juicy. Toasted coconut strips could be used instead of the slivered almonds.

340g/12oz mixture of soft fresh fruit e.g. mango, sharon fruit, banana, dates, papaya, peach, strawberries 2 tbsp stem ginger	4 tbsp slivered almonds 285g/10oz soya or other suitable yogurt mint leaves to decorate

1 Cut the fruit into bite-sized pieces and place in a mixing bowl.
2 Finely dice the ginger and toast the slivered almonds. Set these aside until you are ready to serve the dessert – if you combine all the ingredients at this stage the almonds will soften.
3 Just before serving, mix together the fruit, yogurt, ginger and almonds, saving a few almonds to decorate. Sprinkle the almonds and mint leaves over the dessert and serve immediately.

Summer Fruit Brulée
Serves 2

This refreshing dessert is best made during the summer, when fresh fruit is in season and at its tastiest. Fruits other than those listed can be used but they should be soft and sweet varieties, for example, peach, mango, melon, grapes and bananas. Muscovado sugar can be used instead of the honey if this is acceptable or, if you prefer, you can omit any form of sugar.

225g/8oz fresh or frozen summer fruits e.g. strawberries, raspberries, cherries, blueberries, blackberries 285g/10oz soya or other yogurt	2 tbsp oat or buckwheat flakes (buckwheat is gluten free, oats are not) 2 tsps honey (optional)

1 Mix all the summer fruits and place in two individual, heatproof serving dishes – largish ramekins would be suitable.
2 Pour the yogurt over the fruit.
3 Sprinkle with the flakes then drizzle with the honey. Just before serving, place under a preheated grill and grill until starting to brown. Serve immediately.

Orange and Ginger Flavoured Dried Fruit Salad

Serves 2

I must admit, though the quantities given below are for two, I never make just two servings of this fruit salad, as I adore It. It keeps well for a few days in the fridge and is scrumptious served with porridge or muesli for breakfast. If you don't want to use orange juice, try substituting pineapple or other fruit juices or Earl Grey or jasmine tea. Add a teaspoon of grated lemon rind if desired. This dish does have an intense ginger flavour so reduce the quantity if you wish, and grate the ginger instead of slicing it if you don't want to bite into pieces.

425ml/15fl oz orange juice 2cm/1in piece fresh ginger	170g/6oz mixed dried fruit e.g. apricots, prunes, pears, figs, cherries, cranberries, raisins

1 Place the orange juice in a pan.
2 Peel the ginger, cut it into thin slivers and add it to the orange juice.
3 Add the dried fruit and bring to the boil. Simmer for 20 minutes then allow the fruit to cool. The fruit should be soft and tender. If by any chance it isn't (older fruit can be quite dry) just bring to the boil again and then leave to cool – or, even better, leave it to soak overnight and in the morning it will have plumped up.
4 Serve the fruit warm or cold, just as it is or with yogurt, ice cream, or soya dream (which does contain a little sugar).

Stewed Fresh Pears
with Orange, Ginger and Apricots

Serves 2

I always double the quantity of this recipe and keep it in the fridge for snacks, puddings and breakfast. You can substitute apples for the pears but cook for a few more minutes once the apples are added so that they soften. Pineapple or other fruit juices can be used instead of the orange juice or try using Earl Grey or jasmine tea. Because the ginger is left in pieces, this recipe has quite a kick. Use less ginger or grate it, if you prefer a more subtle flavour.

500ml/18fl oz orange juice	12 dried apricots
2.5cm/1in piece ginger	2 almost ripe medium pears

1 Place the orange juice in a pan.
2 Peel the ginger, cut into thin slivers and add to the orange juice along with the dried apricots. Bring to the boil and simmer for approximately 20 minutes until the ginger and apricots are soft and the orange juice has reduced a little.
3 Peel, core and quarter the pears and add to the pan. Bring to the boil again and simmer for 2 minutes. Remove from the heat and allow the fruit to cool. Keep the pears covered with the juices to prevent them browning.
4 Serve warm or cold with yogurt or ice cream.

Crêpes Bretonnes

Serves 2

Classic crêpes are easy to make from store cupboard ingredients and are ready in minutes. Other fruit could be substituted for the apples – try fresh peaches or apricots or, alternatively, add some sultanas or chopped dried apricots to the apples. The variations are endless.

2 dessert apples	55g/2oz buckwheat flour
approx. 30g/1oz butter or margarine	1 egg
90ml/3fl oz soya or other milk	½ tsp vanilla extract

1 Quarter and core the apples but do not peel. Cut each apple quarter into thin slices.
2 Place a small knob of butter or margarine in a pan and sweat the apples gently until they have softened but not browned. Keep the apples warm.
3 Warm the milk and 15g/½oz butter until the butter is just melted.
4 Process or beat together the milk and butter, flour, egg and vanilla extract. If the batter seems thick, add a little more milk or water until a thin pouring consistency is obtained.
5 Melt a knob of the remaining butter in a 20cm/8in frying pan and pour in sufficient batter to only just cover the base when the pan is tilted from side to side.
6 Sprinkle apple slices over the crêpe then drizzle over a little more batter. Do not cover the apples with batter or the crêpe will be too thick. Cook on a medium heat until golden brown. Turn and cook the other side. Repeat this process with the remaining batter and apples, while keeping the first crêpes warm.
7 Serve warm just as they are or with honey, maple syrup, yogurt or Raspberry Coulis (see page 41).

Banana and Cinnamon Blinis
Serves 2

This is a variation on the Crêpe Bretonnes recipe but the egg white is whisked and the mixture made into little pancakes. Fresh banana is hidden in the blinis as they cook. Other fruit could be substituted for the banana – try blueberries or raspberries and use vanilla extract instead of the cinnamon.

90ml/3fl oz soya or other milk	1 medium egg
approx. 30g/1oz butter or margarine	55g/2oz buckwheat flour
1 banana	½ tsp cinnamon

1 Warm the milk and 15g/½oz of butter until the butter is just melted.
2 Slice the banana.
3 Separate the egg and whisk the egg white until stiff.
4 Process or beat together the milk and butter, flour, egg yolk and cinnamon until well mixed. Fold into the egg white using a metal spoon.
5 Melt a knob of the remaining butter in a 20cm/8in frying pan and pour four separate tablespoons of the batter to form little pancakes. Immediately press three pieces of banana into the surface of each pancake.
6 Cook the blinis until golden brown, then turn over and cook the second side. Keep warm while you repeat the process with the remaining batter.
7 Serve warm just as they are or with honey or maple syrup and yogurt.

Pear and Passion Fruit Sorbet

Serves 2

This is the perfect refreshing summer dessert. In winter, spice it up by adding one tablespoon of chopped stem ginger before serving. You could also use other fruit combinations, such as pineapple and raspberry or peach and strawberry (there's no need to heat the strawberries or raspberries).

2 large ripe pears	4 passion fruit
2 tsps lemon juice	fresh mint leaves to decorate

1   Peel and core the pears and cut into bite-sized pieces. Toss the pieces in the lemon juice to prevent them going brown.
2   Spread the pear pieces out on a baking tray and freeze.
3   Scoop the centres out of the passion fruit and heat to release the juice from the seeds. This will only take a few seconds. Press through a sieve to remove the seeds.
4   Place the passion fruit juice in a food processor, add the frozen pears and process until smooth. It is a good idea to pulse the mixture first to get it started and prevent it trying to escape. If the mixture chops but doesn't become smooth, either add a tablespoon of water or allow the mixture to defrost for 2 minutes. Eventually it will combine into a creamy, smooth sorbet.
5   Serve at once, decorated with the mint leaves.

Fried Bananas in Orange, Coconut and Cinnamon Sauce

Serves 2

These wonderfully sticky, fried bananas are a fun dessert or light snack. Creamed coconut is sold in blocks in the supermarkets and is a really useful store cupboard staple. Other juices could be used instead of the orange juice, such as pineapple.

55g/2oz creamed coconut	2 large bananas
125ml/4fl oz fresh orange juice	1 tsp butter or margarine
1 level tsp grated orange rind	½ tsp cinnamon
1 tsp lemon juice	

1 Cut the creamed coconut into rough chunks and place in a pan with the orange juice, orange rind and lemon juice. Bring to the boil and simmer gently until the coconut has melted to give a smooth creamy sauce.
2 Cut the bananas in half and then in half again lengthwise.
3 Fry the bananas in the butter or margarine until they begin to soften and brown. This will only take a few minutes.
4 Sprinkle with cinnamon and serve immediately, with the orange and coconut sauce.

Creamy Stewed Fruit

Serves 2

What could be simpler than three everyday fruits thrown into a pan and cooked? But it's not what you do – it's the way that you do it. By cutting the banana finely it breaks down to produce a lovely creamy sauce, which is flavoured with orange and cinnamon. You can vary the recipe by using pineapple or mango juice and fresh pears instead of apples.

200ml/7fl oz orange juice	1 large banana
1 level tsp cinnamon	2 dessert apples

1 Place the orange juice and cinnamon in a pan
2 Finely dice the banana and add to the pan. Bring the mixture to the boil and simmer on a low heat until the banana starts to disintegrate, then whisk the mixture to break down the banana completely.
3 Core the apples (don't peel if organic), quarter them and cut the quarters into thin slices.
4 Place these in the pan, bring the mixture to the boil and simmer on a low heat, stirring occasionally, for 10–15 minutes until the apples are just cooked.
5 Serve the fruit warm, with cold soya dream (this contains a little sugar), yogurt or ice cream.

Baked Apple Custard

Serves 3–4

In this variation on a traditional egg custard, dates, rather than sugar, are used to add sweetness. Serve decorated with some fresh fruit, such as strawberries or blueberries, and with some cold yogurt if desired.

2 dessert apples	285ml/10fl oz soya or other milk
60ml/2fl oz water	½ tsp vanilla extract
55g/2oz chopped dates	30g/1oz ground almonds
2 medium eggs	grated nutmeg

1 Set the oven temperature to 170°C/325°F/Gas Mark 3 and grease a 20–22cm/8–9in flan dish.
2 Peel and core the apples and cut the flesh into small pieces. Place in a pan with the water and dates, cover and simmer gently until the apples and dates are soft. Allow to cool.
3 Place the eggs, milk, vanilla extract and ground almonds in a processor. Add the cooled apple and date mixture and process until smooth.
4 Place the mixture in the flan dish and sprinkle with nutmeg. Bake the custard in the oven for approximately 30 minutes until the custard is just set. Do not over-cook or the custard will start to curdle.
5 Serve warm or cold.

Baked Apricot Custard

Cut 115g/4oz of dried apricots into small pieces and simmer in 125ml/4fl oz of water until the apricots are soft and the water has been absorbed. Process these until they are smooth. Use in the previous recipe instead of the apples, water and dates and add 3 drops of almond extract instead of the vanilla extract.

Baked Custard Tart

Serves 4

To produce the custard tart pictured on the front cover, make up half the quantity of the Nutty Flapjack recipe from page 194 and press into a 20cm/8in, deep flan dish. Bake blind for 12 minutes at 170°C/325°F/Gas Mark 3. Make up half the quantity of the baked apple custard recipe and pour into the tart case. Bake for approximately 25 minutes or until the custard is just set.

Coconut and Cardamom Rice with Mango Sauce

Serves 2

This rich creamy rice dessert is a really comforting treat on cold winter's days. It is an Indian version of a traditional rice pudding but, as it's made with rice flakes, it is a quick and easy alternative. Passion fruit makes a delicious addition to the mango sauce. If using, process with the mango and then sieve the sauce to remove the seeds. Decorate with toasted coconut strips instead of the pistachios if desired.

85g/3oz rice flakes	400ml/14fl oz boiling water
200ml/7fl oz coconut milk	1 medium ripe mango
½ tsp cardamom powder	1 tbsp pistachio nuts to decorate
30g/1oz chopped dates	

1 Place the rice flakes in a pan with the coconut milk, cardamom, chopped dates and boiling water.
2 Bring to the boil and simmer for approximately 20 minutes until the rice is thick and creamy. Beat the mixture to break up the dates.
3 Peel and stone the mango. Cube half of the flesh. Process the remaining mango to produce a smooth sauce, adding a little water if the sauce is too thick.
4 Place the warm rice pudding in ramekin-type dishes, decorate with the pistachio nuts and serve on plates, accompanied by the mango and mango sauce.

Rhubarb and Banana Ice Cream
Serves 2

I was really tempted to make this a rhubarb and ginger ice cream but I managed to stop myself. I just adore ginger in any form and I'm inclined to add it to every recipe. It does, however, go well with this one, so add 1 tablespoon of chopped stem ginger if you like the taste and can cope with the small amount of added sugar. I always double up on the rhubarb and date mixture and freeze some for another day.

285g/10oz rhubarb	½ tsp vanilla extract
30ml/1fl oz water	2 medium bananas
55g/2oz chopped dates	chopped nuts to decorate

1 Cut the rhubarb into 2cm/¾in pieces, place in a pan and cover with cold water. Bring to the boil, but as soon as the water comes to the boil sieve the rhubarb. This process removes some of the sharpness of the rhubarb.
2 Place the sieved rhubarb back in the pan and add the 30ml/1fl oz of water and the chopped dates. Cover and simmer gently on a low heat until the rhubarb and dates are soft. Allow to cool.
3 Place the rhubarb mixture in ice cube trays and freeze until solid.
4 Put the frozen rhubarb in a food processor along with the vanilla extract. Roughly chop the bananas and add to the processor. Process until smooth. It's a good idea to pulse the mixture first until it starts combining to prevent it trying to escape.
5 Serve at once, decorated with chopped nuts and some chopped ginger if desired.

Pineapple, Mango
and Coconut Ice Cream

Serves 2

I find it useful to keep extra fruit in the freezer for when I need a speedy dessert. I also love to make ice cream for a mid-afternoon snack on a hot summer's day, and it's so easy when the ingredients are already there in the freezer. Peaches make a good substitute for the mango in this recipe.

170g/6oz fresh pineapple	fresh fruit and/or toasted coconut strips
170g/6oz fresh mango	to decorate
285ml/10fl oz coconut milk	

1 Cube the pineapple and mango flesh and spread the pieces out on a baking tray. Freeze until solid.
2 Place the frozen fruit pieces in a processor with the coconut milk and process until smooth. It is a good idea to pulse the mixture to help it to combine and prevent it trying to escape.
3 Serve at once, decorated with some fresh fruit and toasted coconut.

Fresh Fruit Fondue
with Raspberry Sauce

Serves 2

This simple but delightful dessert is the perfect ending for an informal meal. Serve the raspberry sauce in individual ramekins and the fruit alongside so that each person can use a fork to dip the fruit into their portion of sauce. The peach helps to thicken the raspberry sauce but it could be omitted or replaced with other fruit, such as mango or banana.

RASPBERRY SAUCE:	455g/1lb selection of fruit, choose
225g/8oz raspberries (fresh or frozen)	from pineapple, peach, apricots,
1 ripe peach	mango, strawberries, banana, sharon
1 teaspoon honey (optional)	fruit, plums, apple, papaya

1 To make the sauce, stone the peach, process it with the raspberries and honey then press the mixture through a sieve to remove the raspberry seeds and peach skin.
2 Cut the fruit selection into bite-sized pieces and place on two plates. Serve the raspberry sauce in ramekins or small dishes alongside the fruit.
3 Chill for 20 minutes or serve at room temperature.

Fresh Fruit Fondue
with Carob Chocolate Sauce

Serves 2

This is a heavenly version of the previous recipe. Here, cold fresh fruit is served ready to dip into a mouthwatering carob chocolate sauce. It's hard to believe that easy, healthy cooking can be this simple or delicious. Just make up the carob sauce and serve instead of the raspberry sauce as before. For a source of good quality carob chocolate, see the list of suppliers at the back of this book. Alternatively, you could use Green and Blacks organic, which is dairy free but not sugar free.

CAROB SAUCE:	455g/1lb selection of fruit, choose
55g/2oz chopped dried dates	from pineapple, peach, apricots,
60ml/2fl oz water	mango, strawberries, banana, sharon
55g/2oz carob chocolate	fruit, plums, apple, papaya
125ml/4fl oz soya or other milk	

1 Place the dates and water in a small pan and simmer on a low heat until the dates have softened and most of the water has been absorbed.
2 Break the chocolate into small pieces, add to the dates in the pan and allow the chocolate to melt. Remove from the heat.
3 Process or beat together the milk and the chocolate mixture until the sauce is smooth and creamy. Pour into two ramekin-type dishes and cool. The sauce will thicken as the chocolate sets.
4 Serve with chunks of fresh fruit to dip.

Apricot and Yogurt Fruit Swirl

Serves 2

This dessert is simplicity itself, made in minutes from ingredients that I always have at hand. If you want a richer, creamier dessert you could use half yogurt and half soya dream, though this does contain a little sugar.

400g tin apricot halves in fruit juice	2 tbsp toasted slivered almonds
225g/8oz soya or other yogurt	

1   Drain the apricots and discard the juice. Process the fruit until smooth
2   Layer the apricots and yogurt in sundae glasses, finishing with an apricot layer.
3   Using a spoon, stir the two layers together just enough to create a swirling, two-tone effect.
4   Sprinkle over the toasted almonds and serve chilled.

Carob Chocolate and Orange Mousse

Serves 2

At times, we all feel like some indulgent comfort food. Well this pudding fits the bill, but instead of being bad for you it's full of good ingredients. Carob chocolate varies tremendously, especially when it's sugar free, and some of them I find unacceptable. The manufacturer of the one I used is listed at the back of the book. You could also use Green and Blacks organic chocolate, which is dairy free but not sugar free. Molasses contains the goodness left over from sugar manufacturing and is full of vitamins and minerals. It does, however, contain a little sugar so it can be omitted if you prefer.

1 dsp molasses	grated rind ½ orange
60ml/2fl oz orange juice	2 egg whites
55g/2oz carob chocolate	chopped nuts to decorate
170g/6oz silken tofu	

1 In a small bowl, blend the molasses with the orange juice. Break the carob chocolate into small pieces and add to the mixture.
2 Place the bowl over a pan of simmering water until the chocolate has melted. Allow to cool a little.
3 Process or beat the silken tofu and the orange rind until smooth and creamy, then add the carob mixture and blend.
4 In a clean bowl, whisk the egg whites until stiff and then fold in the carob mixture using a metal spoon.
5 Place the mixture into two serving glasses and chill (the mousse can be made ahead of time and kept in the fridge overnight). Decorate with chopped nuts and serve.

Banana and Mango Crème Pots
Serves 2

This rich and creamy dessert is a really comforting treat. You can make it with other fruit as well as mango – try peach, sharon fruit or cherries.

1 medium ripe mango	2 level tsp corn or rice flour
1 medium banana	400ml/14fl oz soya or other milk
2 egg yolks	1 tsp honey (optional)
½ tsp vanilla extract	2 sprigs mint

1 Peel and stone the mango and cut the flesh into small pieces. Place the mango flesh in the base of two largish ramekin dishes, saving a few pieces to decorate.
2 Process the banana, egg yolks, vanilla and flour until smooth. Add the milk and honey and mix well.
3 Place the mixture in a pan and heat gently, stirring until thick and just starting to boil. Remove the pan from the heat immediately and allow the mixture to cool a little.
4 Pour the crème mixture over the mango in the pots and chill. Serve the pots decorated with the remaining mango slices and mint.

Raspberry Cream Crowdie
Serves 2

This recipe is based on a traditional Scottish pudding, which uses oatmeal rather than the hazelnuts used here. Try the traditional recipe if you can tolerate gluten as it really does taste delightful, but then so does the hazelnut version. Use medium oatmeal and toast it in the oven until golden brown.

55g/2oz hazelnuts	1 tbsp runny honey (optional)
285g/10oz soya or other yogurt	225g/8oz fresh or frozen raspberries

1 Toast the hazelnuts in a hot oven or under the grill until golden brown. Rub off the skins. Process the nuts until they are finely chopped.
2 Combine the hazelnuts, soya yogurt and honey.
3 Reserve a few raspberries for decoration then place alternate layers of raspberries and yogurt mixture in two tall sundae glasses. Decorate with the remaining raspberries. Serve immediately or the nuts will soften.

Apple Cream Crowdie

Stew 2 large dessert apples with ½ teaspoon of cinnamon and use instead of the raspberries in the above recipe.

Almond and Carob Torte
Serves 2–3

As carob tortes go, this is a pretty foolproof version and one that produces a really moist and yummy feast. Why not double the quantity and make extra? It keeps well in the fridge for 2–3 days but also freezes fine. If you do not like carob flour then substitute sugar-free cocoa powder.

55g/2oz chopped dried dates	2 medium eggs, separated
60ml/2fl oz water	30g/1oz carob flour
55g/2oz butter or margarine	1 level dsp molasses (optional)
55g/2oz almonds	½ tsp vanilla extract

1 Grease and line a 15cm/6in loose-bottomed cake tin and set the oven temperature to 180°C/350°F/Gas Mark 4
2 Place the dates and water in a pan and simmer on a low heat until the dates are soft and the water has been absorbed.
3 Remove the pan from the heat. Cut the butter or margarine into small pieces and add to the pan. Allow this to melt in the heat from the dates.
4 Process the almonds until fairly finely chopped, but not ground, and remove them from the processor.
5 Process the dates and butter, egg yolks, carob flour, molasses and vanilla extract. Add the almonds and process until combined.
6 Beat the egg whites in a large bowl until stiff then fold in the carob mixture using a metal spoon.
7 Spread the mixture into the prepared tin and bake on the middle shelf of the oven until spongy when pressed. This will take approximately 40 minutes.
8 Cool in the tin and then remove and serve with a little yogurt, ice cream or soya dream (this does contain a little sugar) and some fresh fruit, such as strawberries, raspberries, blueberries or pears.

Fresh Figs with Yogurt, Mint and Orange
Serves 2

This is such a simple dessert but it's so delicious that you will want to serve it again and again. I first served it with fresh figs picked straight from the garden on a summer's day – and it made the hard work of gardening worthwhile.

3 figs	6 heaped tbsp soya or other yogurt
2 tbsp freshly squeezed orange juice	2 tsp honey (optional)
1 tsp grated orange rind	mint leaves to decorate
1 tbsp chopped fresh mint	

1   Cut the figs in half and place in serving bowls. Drizzle with the orange juice.
2   Mix together the orange rind, mint and the yogurt and spoon into the bowls next to the figs. Allow to stand for 15 minutes to allow the flavours to combine.
3   Drizzle with the honey if using, decorate with the mint leaves and serve.

Cakes and Biscuits

It is impossible to make biscuits and cakes without some form of sweetener and/or some fat. I have tried to use as little fat and sugar substitute as possible in these recipes while still making tasty treats, but I have also tried to include as much goodness as possible – in the form of nuts, seeds, fresh and dried fruit, and flakes and flours. I use butter when cooking as I prefer the taste, but margarine is quite acceptable, provided it is one of the non-hydrogenated ones. I use dates as a sugar substitute as these are an unprocessed form of sweetener that still contains all its fibre and nutriments. If these are not acceptable then you could try substituting another dried fruit or, failing that, some stewed apple or mashed banana.

I have tried, where possible, to use a proprietary gluten-free flour to make buying and cooking easier (see list of suppliers), but I have also tried most recipes using rice flour in case some of the ingredients in the gluten-free flour are not acceptable. Gluten-free baking powder is readily available in health food shops.

If you use an egg replacer in recipes, add an extra half a teaspoon of baking powder as cakes don't rise as well with this as they do with eggs.

Because the biscuits and cakes do not contain a lot of fat and sugar they do not keep as well as traditional cakes, therefore I recommend freezing any excess. It's also wonderful to have cakes and cookies frozen for when you feel like a treat or if guests arrive unexpectedly.

If your processor has a plastic blade, use this for these recipes, as it prevents nuts and dried fruit from being broken up too much.

Nutty Flapjacks
Makes 12

I originally made these flapjacks with oats but they are equally delicious with buckwheat or rye flakes. They are also very simple to make. Blackstrap molasses contains the goodness leftover from the sugar cane when sugar is made. It is full of vitamins and minerals, though it does contain a little sugar residue. Leave out the molasses, honey or maple syrup in the flapjack recipes if you cannot tolerate any sugar. The flapjacks will still be acceptable though a little more crumbly.

115g/4oz chopped dried dates	55g/2oz sunflower seeds
90ml/3fl oz water	225g/8oz oat, rye or buckwheat
115g/4oz butter or margarine	flakes (buckwheat is gluten free, oats
2 tbsp blackstrap molasses	and rye are not)
55g/2oz almonds	

1   Set the oven temperature to 200°C/400°F/Gas Mark 6.
2   Place the dates and water in a pan and simmer on a low heat until the dates are soft and most of the water has been absorbed.
3   Add the butter or margarine and molasses and continue to heat until melted. Beat well to break up the dates.
4   Cut the almonds into small pieces and add to the pan along with the sunflower seeds and flakes. Stir well to combine.
5   Spread the mixture onto an ungreased baking tray (approx. 20 x 30cm/8 x 12in) and press down well.
6   Bake for approximately 20 minutes or until the flapjacks are firm and brown.
7   Cut into 12 slices while still warm and then leave to cool in the tin. Store in an airtight container and eat within 3 days or freeze.

Nutty Flapjacks with Walnuts, Apricots and Maple Syrup

Follow the previous recipe but use walnuts or pecans instead of almonds, chopped dried apricots instead of sunflower seeds and maple syrup instead of molasses – delicious.

Nutty Flapjacks with Pine Nuts, Honey and Ginger

Substitute 30g/1oz of pine nuts, 30g/1oz of sunflower seeds and 55g/2oz chopped crystallized ginger (which does contain a little sugar) for the nuts and seeds in the main recipe. Instead of molasses, use honey.

Nutty Flapjacks with Dried Cranberries and Cashew Nuts

Substitute dried cranberries and cashew nuts for the almonds and sunflower seeds and use honey or maple syrup to sweeten.

Nutty Flapjacks with Dried Cherry, Almonds and Sesame Seeds

Use dried cherries instead of sunflower seeds and sprinkle 2 tablespoons of sesame seeds over the surface. Press in well before baking.

Nutty Flapjacks with Coconut and Cinnamon

Replace the sunflower seeds with chopped coconut chips and the molasses with honey, and add 1 teaspoon of cinnamon.

Apricot Slices
Makes 12

In these yummy slices, moist apricots sit between two layers of crumbly biscuit. The molasses can be omitted if you cannot tolerate any sugar, though molasses does contain lots of goodness as well as a little sugar.

285g/10oz dried apricots	115g/4oz gluten-free flour (or rice flour)
180ml/6fl oz water	
1 tsp lemon rind	1 tsp cinnamon
115g/4oz butter or margarine	225g/8oz oat or buckwheat flakes
1 tbsp molasses	(buckwheat is gluten free, oats are not)
	55g/2oz sunflower seeds

1   Set the oven temperature to 200°C/400°F/Gas Mark 6.
2   Finely dice the apricots, place in a pan and add the water. Simmer on a low heat until they are soft and most of the water has been absorbed. Mash or process the apricots with the lemon rind until they are fairly smooth. Add a little water if the mixture is too stiff to spread easily.
3   Place the butter or margarine and the molasses in a medium sized pan and melt over a low heat.
4   Add the flour, cinnamon, flakes, sunflower seeds and two tablespoons of the apricot mixture. Mix by hand until crumbly and combined.
5   Spread half the flour and flake mixture in an ungreased Swiss roll tin (approximately 18 x 28cm/7 x 11in) and press down firmly. Spread the apricot mixture over this then cover it with the remaining oat mix. Press well by hand to flatten and firm.
6   Bake the slices for 20–25 minutes until firm and golden brown. Cut into 12 squares while warm and allow the slices to cool in the tin. Store in an airtight container and eat within 3 days or freeze.

Date Slices

Follow the recipe for apricot slices but substitute chopped dates for the apricots.

Fig and Orange Slices

Follow the recipe for apricot slices but substitute dried figs for the apricots and use orange rind instead of the lemon rind. The water can also be replaced with orange juice for a more intense orange flavour.

Walnut and Raisin Cookies
Makes 14

I always like to have some home-baked goodies in the freezer, as part of me loves the tradition of afternoon tea. It makes a lovely interlude to summer gardening and cheers up a miserable winter day. These cookies are ideal, as they don't take long to defrost.

55g/2oz walnuts	85g/3oz gluten-free flour (or rice flour)
115g/4oz softened butter or	140g/5oz oat or buckwheat flakes
margarine	(buckwheat is gluten free, oats are not)
1 tbsp honey (optional)	55g/2oz raisins
1 tsp ground mixed spice	extra flakes for coating
1 medium egg or egg replacer	

1 Set the oven temperature to 180°C/350°F/Gas Mark 4.
2 Finely chop the walnuts.
3 Process the butter, honey, mixed spice, egg and flour until well mixed.
4 Add the walnuts, flakes and raisins and process for a few seconds to combine. Do not over-process or you will break up the nuts and raisins.
5 Roll the mixture into walnut-sized balls and then roll in the extra flakes to coat. Place on an ungreased baking tray and, using the back of a fork, flatten to make biscuit shapes about 5mm/¼in thick.
6 Bake for approximately 12 minutes or until golden brown.
7 Allow the biscuits to cool on the tray for 5 minutes then place them on a wire cooling rack. Once cold, store in an airtight tin and eat within three days or freeze.

Chewy Fruit and Nut Cookies
Makes 12

These chewy biscuits are not only great to eat but they are packed full of so much goodness that you really are doing yourself a favour by eating them.

55g/2oz chopped dried dates	55g/2oz ground almonds
60ml/2fl oz water	55g/2oz sultanas
85g/3oz butter or margarine	140g/5oz chopped coconut chips
1 tbsp honey (optional)	30g/1oz sunflower seeds
140g/5oz oat, rye or buckwheat flakes (buckwheat is gluten free, oats and rye are not)	55g/2oz chopped almonds
	1 tsp cinnamon
55g/2oz gluten-free flour (or rice flour)	1 medium egg or egg replacer

1   Set the oven temperature to 180°C/350°F/Gas Mark 4.
2   Place the chopped dates and water in a pan and simmer over a low heat until soft. Add the butter and honey, allow them to melt then whisk to combine.
3   Add the flakes, flour, ground almonds, sultanas, coconut chips, sunflower seeds, chopped almonds and cinnamon and mix well. Beat the egg and combine with the rest of the ingredients.
4   Using floured hands, roll the mixture into walnut-sized balls, place on a greased baking sheet and press into thick biscuit shapes.
5   Bake for approximately 20 minutes or until golden brown and firm to touch.
6   Allow the cookies to cool for 5 minutes on the tray then place on a wire rack. Once cold, store in an airtight container and eat within 3 days or freeze.

Peanut Butter and Raisin Cookies

Makes 16

These cookies were labelled 'ever so scrumptious' by a friend who tested them. She had to hide them from her husband to stop him eating them all.

85g/3oz chopped dried dates	85g/3oz gluten-free flour (or rice flour)
60ml/2fl oz water	115g/4oz oat or buckwheat flakes
85g/3oz butter or margarine	(buckwheat is gluten free, oats are not)
115g/4oz smooth peanut butter	55g/2oz raisins
½ tsp vanilla extract	85g/3oz salted peanuts

1   Set the oven temperature to 180°C/350°F/Gas Mark 4.
2   Place the dates and water in a pan and simmer on a low heat until they are soft and most of the water has been absorbed. Remove the pan from the heat. Cut the butter or margarine into small pieces, add it to the pan and allow it to melt.
3   Process the date and butter mixture until smooth and creamy. Add the peanut butter, vanilla extract, flour and the flakes and process until well mixed.
4   Add the raisins and peanuts and process for a few seconds to combine. Do not over-process or the nuts and raisins will break up.
5   Roll the mixture into balls the size of a small egg and place on an ungreased baking tray. Flatten into biscuit shapes using the back of a fork.
6   Bake the biscuits for approximately 10–15 minutes until golden brown.
7   Leave the biscuits to cool on the tray for 5 minutes then transfer to a wire rack. Store in an airtight container once cool. Eat within 3 days or freeze.

Carob and Brazil Nut Shortbread
Makes 8

Brazil nuts and carob combine well in this very crisp shortbread. The molasses can be omitted if you cannot tolerate even the smallest amount of sugar. The recipe works best if the butter or margarine is really cold. Use it straight from the fridge or freeze it for 10 minutes before using.

85g/3oz Brazil nuts	55g/2oz soya or gram flour
85g/3oz butter or margarine	1 tbsp molasses
55g/2oz carob flour	½ tsp vanilla extract
55g/2oz ground almonds	

1　Set the oven temperature to 150°C/300°F/Gas Mark 2.
2　Cut each whole Brazil nut into three or four pieces.
3　Cut the butter or margarine into small pieces and process with the carob flour, ground almonds, flour, molasses and vanilla extract until it forms a fine breadcrumb-like texture. Be careful not to over-process or the mixture will bind together before you have added the next ingredient.
4　Tip the mixture into a bowl and add the Brazil nuts. Use your hand to combine the ingredients and then press the mixture into an ungreased 18–20cm/7–8in sandwich tin.
5　Bake for approximately 25 minutes or until the Brazil nuts are brown and the shortbread is firm to touch.
6　Cut the shortbread into wedges while it is still warm and allow them to cool in the tin. Store in an airtight container when cool and eat within 3 days or freeze.

Flakemeal Shorties

Makes 16

The butter or margarine needs to be very cold in this recipe. Use straight from the fridge or place in the freezer for 10 minutes to cool. Leave out the honey if you cannot tolerate anything sweet. The recipe will still work but the shorties will be less sweet.

115g/4oz cashews	1 tsp vanilla extract
115g/4oz soya or gram flour	1 tbsp honey (optional)
1 rounded tsp cinnamon	115g/4oz oat or buckwheat flakes
115g/4oz butter or margarine	(buckwheat is gluten free, oats are not)

1   Set the oven temperature to 150°C/300°F/Gas Mark 2.
2   Process the cashew nuts until finely ground.
3   Add the flour and cinnamon. Cut the butter or margarine into small pieces and add this to the processor.
4   Process again until the mixture resembles fine breadcrumbs. Be careful not to over-process or the mixture will bind together before you have added the next ingredients.
5   Add the honey and vanilla extract and process until the mixture combines.
6   Spread half of the flakes onto a work surface and place the shortcake mixture on top. Using the remaining flakes to prevent the mixture sticking, roll out to approximately 5mm/¼in thickness. Most of the flakes should be attached to the shorties by the time they are rolled out.
7   Cut the shortcake mixture into rounds and place these on an ungreased baking sheet. Bake for approximately 10–15 minutes until brown around the edges.
8   Allow the biscuits to cool on the tray for a few minutes then transfer to a wire rack to cool completely. Store in an airtight tin and eat within 3 days or freeze.

Banana and Walnut Wedges

Makes 8

This recipe produces a delicious spongy biscuit that is quite sweet because of the added fruit.

55g/2oz butter or margarine	55g/2oz walnuts
1 eating apple	55g/2oz desiccated coconut
225g/8oz bananas (weighed after peeling)	55g/2oz oat or buckwheat flakes (buckwheat is gluten free, oats are not)
½ tsp vanilla extract	1 tbsp extra flakes to sprinkle over
1 tsp mixed spice	

1 Set the oven temperature to 200°C/400°F/Gas Mark 6 and grease a 23cm/9in round sandwich tin.
2 Melt the butter or margarine.
3 Peel, quarter and core the apple and process with the butter or margarine, bananas, vanilla extract and mixed spice until smooth and creamy.
4 Add the walnuts, the coconut and the flakes and process until the mixture is combined and the walnuts have broken up a little.
5 Place in the sandwich tin, level the surface and sprinkle over the extra flakes.
6 Bake for approximately 25 minutes or until firm to the touch and golden brown. Cut into wedges while they are still warm and allow to cool for 5 minutes in the tin before placing on a wire cooling rack.
7 Store in an airtight tin when cold and eat within 3 days or freeze.

Country Apple Cake

Chunks of apple and plump, succulent sultanas add sweetness to this moist cake. It is delicious eaten warm or cold and can be served as a pudding with custard or soya dream (this contains a little sugar).

115g/4oz chopped dried dates	170g/6oz gluten-free flour (or rice flour)
90ml/3fl oz water	2 rounded tsp mixed spice
170g/6oz sharp eating apples (weighed after preparing)	2 rounded tsp baking powder
115g/4oz butter or margarine	115g/4oz sultanas
2 medium eggs	

1   Grease and line a 15–18cm/6–7in, deep-sided cake tin. Set the oven temperature to 170°C/325°F/Gas Mark 3.
2   Place the dates and water in a pan and simmer over a low heat until they are soft and most of the water has been absorbed. Allow them to cool a little.
3   Peel and core the apples and cut the flesh into small pieces by hand.
4   Process the dates and butter or margarine until creamy. Add the eggs, flour, spice and baking powder and process to combine.
5   Add the apples and sultanas and process for a few seconds to combine. Do not over-process at this stage or the fruit will break up. The mixture should have a soft dropping consistency. Add a little milk or water if it is too stiff.
6   Place the mixture into the cake tin and bake for 50–60 minutes or until golden brown and firm to the touch.
7   Allow the cake to cool for 5 minutes in the tin then turn out onto a wire cooling rack and peel off the lining paper. Store in an airtight container once cold and eat within 3 days or freeze.

Lemon Polenta Cake

Lemon polenta cake makes a good dessert, served slightly warm with some fresh blueberries, raspberries or strawberries and some yogurt, ice cream or soya dream (which contains a little sugar). If you cannot tolerate corn, use ground rice instead of the polenta. This is readily available in Asian shops.

115g/4oz chopped dried dates	55g/2oz polenta
90ml/3fl oz water	55g/2oz gluten-free flour (or rice flour)
115g/4oz butter or margarine	1 rounded tsp baking powder
2 medium eggs or egg replacer	2 tsps grated lemon rind
85g/3oz ground almonds	2 tbsp lemon juice

1   Grease and line a 455g/1lb loaf tin or 18–20cm/6–7in sandwich tin and set the oven temperature to 180°C/350°F/Gas Mark 4.
2   Place the dates and water in a pan and simmer over a low heat until they are soft and most of the water has been absorbed. Allow them to cool a little.
3   Process the dates and butter or margarine until creamy.
4   Add the eggs, ground almonds, polenta, flour, baking powder, lemon rind and lemon juice. Process until well combined. The mixture should have a soft dropping consistency, so add a little extra water if needed.
5   Place the mixture in the baking tin and bake for approximately 45 minutes or until golden brown and firm to the touch.
6   Allow the cake to cool in the tin for 5 minutes then turn out onto a wire rack and remove the lining paper. Once cold, store in an airtight container and eat within three days or freeze.

Raisin and Almond Cake

The ground almonds in this cake keep it really moist, while the polenta provides a wonderful texture. Try using ground rice (available in Asian shops) instead of the polenta, and rice flour instead of the gluten-free flour if these are not acceptable. Cashew nuts can be ground and used instead of the ground almonds.

115g/4oz chopped dried dates	50g/1½oz polenta
90ml/3fl oz water	50g/1½oz gluten-free flour (or rice
115g/4oz butter or margarine	flour)
2 medium eggs or egg replacer	1 rounded tsp baking powder
3 drops almond extract	85g/3oz raisins
85g/3 oz ground almonds	

1 Grease and line a 455g/1lb loaf tin or 18–20cm/6–7in sandwich tin and set the oven temperature to 180°C/350°F/Gas Mark 4.
2 Place the dates and water in a pan and simmer over a low heat until they are soft and most of the water has been absorbed. Allow them to cool.
3 Process the dates and butter or margarine until creamy.
4 Add the eggs, almond extract, ground almonds, polenta, flour and baking powder and process until well mixed.
5 Add the raisins and process briefly to combine. The mixture should have a soft dropping consistency, so add a little extra water if needed but don't overprocess or the fruit will break up.
6 Place the mixture in the prepared tin and bake for approximately 50 minutes or until golden brown and firm to the touch.
7 Allow the cake to cool in the tin for 5 minutes then turn out onto a wire rack and remove the lining paper. Once cold, store in an airtight container and eat within three days or freeze.

Rhubarb and Vanilla Cake

The flavours of rhubarb and vanilla combine exceptionally well in this unusual but scrumptious cake. Try serving it warm as a dessert, with some rhubarb ice cream or soya dream (which does contain a little sugar). To make a rhubarb and ginger cake, fold in 55g/2oz of chopped crystallized or stem ginger before baking.

115g/4oz rhubarb	125g/4½oz gluten-free flour (or rice
115g/4oz chopped dried dates	flour)
60ml/2fl oz water	2 medium eggs
125g/4½oz butter or margarine	2 level tsp baking powder
	1 tsp vanilla extract

1 Grease and line a 455g/1lb loaf tin or a 15cm/6in sandwich tin and set the oven temperature to 180°C/350°F/Gas Mark 4.
2 Slice the rhubarb and place in a pan with the chopped dates and water. Bring to the boil then cover and simmer on the lowest heat until the rhubarb and dates are soft and mushy and most of the water has been absorbed. Allow to cool.
3 Process the rhubarb mixture with the butter or margarine until smooth and creamy. Add the flour, eggs, baking powder and vanilla extract and process again. The mixture should have a soft dropping consistency, so add a little extra water if needed.
4 Place the mixture in the baking tin and bake for approximately 45 minutes or until golden brown and spongy to touch.
5 Allow the cake to cool in the tin for 5 minutes then turn out onto a wire rack and remove the lining paper. Once cold, store in an airtight container and eat within 3 days or freeze.

Fruit and Nut Tea Bread

This fat-free tea bread is packed full of goodness. It's delicious served warm, or sliced and buttered when cool. I cut any surplus into slices and freeze it. It's easy then to defrost a slice whenever you feel like a treat. You can vary this tea bread by substituting different fruits and nuts. Candied peel contains a little sugar so you may want to use some dried cherries or cranberries instead.

55g/2oz chopped dried dates	55g/2oz candied peel
60ml/2fl oz water	85g/3oz gluten free flour (or rice flour)
55g/2oz dried apricots	1 rounded tsp baking powder
55g/2oz walnuts	1 rounded tsp mixed spice
30g/1oz sunflower seeds	1 medium egg or egg substitute
55g/2oz sultanas	60ml/2fl oz milk

1 Grease and line a 455g/1lb loaf tin and set the oven temperature to 180°C/350°F/Gas Mark 4.
2 Place the dates and water in a pan and simmer on a low heat until they are soft and most of the water has been absorbed.
3 Cut the apricots and walnuts into small pieces and place in a bowl with the sunflower seeds, sultanas and candied peel.
4 Process the dates, flour, baking powder, mixed spice, egg and milk until well mixed. The mixture should have a soft dropping consistency, so add a little extra milk if needed, but do not overprocess or the fruit and nuts will break up.
5 Add the nuts and fruit and process for a few seconds to combine.
6 Place the mixture in the loaf tin and bake for approximately 40–50 minutes until firm to the touch.
7 Allow the tea bread to cool for 5 minutes in the tin, then turn out onto a wire rack and remove the lining paper. Once cold, store in an airtight container and eat within 3 days or freeze.

Cranberry, Apricot and Sultana Loaf

This recipe produces a good textured fat-free loaf, which rises well and tastes wonderful sliced and spread with butter or margarine. Try variations on this loaf – replace the apricots with prunes or figs and use cherries instead of the cranberries.

55g/2oz chopped dried dates	1 heaped tsp mixed spice
45ml/1½fl oz water	1 level tsp bicarbonate of soda
140g/5oz soya or other yogurt	55g/2oz dried chopped apricots
1 medium egg	55g/2oz dried cranberries
125g/4½oz gluten-free flour (or rice flour)	30g/1oz sultanas

1 Set the oven temperature to 180°C/350°F/Gas Mark 4 and grease and line a 455g/1lb loaf tin.
2 Simmer the chopped dates in the water, over a low heat, until they are soft and most of the water has been absorbed. Allow them to cool a little.
3 Process the dates, yogurt, egg, flour, mixed spice and bicarbonate of soda until well mixed.
4 Add the dried apricots, cranberries and sultanas and process for a few seconds to combine. The mixture should have a soft dropping consistency, so add a little extra water if needed, but do not overprocess or the fruit will break up.
5 Place the mixture in the loaf tin and bake for approximately 30–35 minutes or until brown and firm to touch.
6 Cool for 5 minutes in the tin, then place on a wire cooling rack and remove the lining paper.
7 Once cold, store in an airtight tin and eat within 3 days or freeze in slices.

Resources

Belazu

7 Barretts Green Road, London NW10 7AE

Tel: 02088 389670

Fax: 02088 381913

Email: info@belazu.com

Website: www.belazu.com

Suppliers of the pickled lemons used in these recipes

Tiger Tiger

Bull Close Road, Lenton Industrial Estate, Nottingham NG7 2UT

Tel: 0115 985 1300

Fax: 0115 985 1302

Email: tmetson@tiger-tiger.co.uk

Website: www.tigertiger.info

Suppliers of fish sauce with only 2% sugar and no additives

D&D Chocolates Ltd

Centenary Business Centre, Hammond Close, Attleborough Fields, Nuneaton, Warwickshire CV11 6RY

Tel and Fax: 02476 370 909

Email: contact@d-dchocolates.com

Website: www.d-dchocolates.com

Suppliers of sugar- and dairy-free carob chocolate

Natco Foods Ltd
Osier Way, Swan Business Park, Buckingham MK18 1TB
Email: info@natcofoods.com
Website: www.natco-online.com

Suppliers of tamarind concentrate without additives

Kitchen Garden Organics
Waverley Centre, Coventry Road, Cubbington, Warwickshire CW32 7UJ
Tel: 01926 851989
Fax: 01926 851997
Email: manager@kitchen-garden.co.uk
Website: www.kitchen-garden.co.uk.

Suppliers of salt-pickled, dairy-free horseradish and also organic herbs and
spices

The Organic Herb Trading Company
Court Farm, Milverton, Somerset TA4 1NF
Tel: 01823 401205
Fax: 01823 401001
Email: info@organicherbtrading.com
Website: www.organicherbtrading.com

Suppliers of organic herbs and spices, including pure mustard powder

Doves Farm Foods

Salisbury Road, Hungerford, Berkshire RG17 0RF

Tel: 01488 684880

Fax: 01488 685235

Email: cmarraige@dovesfarm.co.uk

Website: www.dovesfarm.co.uk

Suppliers of the gluten-free flour used in some recipes

Suma Foods

Lacy Way, Lowfields Business Park, Elland, Yorkshire HX5 9DB

Tel: 0845 458 2290

Fax: 0845 4582294

Email: Info@suma.coop

Website: www.suma.coop

Suppliers of natural foods to shops, they will also deliver to individuals if there is no local outlet

Swinton Health Foods

177 Moorside Road, Swinton, Manchester M27 9LD

Tel: 0161 793 0091

Fax: 0161 728 6087

Email: swintonhealthfoods@ukonline.co.uk

Provides mail order for supplements, specialist foods and books

British Association for Nutritional Therapy (BANT)
27 Old Gloucester Street, London WC1N 3XX
Tel and Fax: 08706 061284
Email: theadministrator@bant.org.uk
Website: www.bant.org.uk

The professional body for nutritional therapists – contact to find a therapist
in your area

The Institute for Optimum Nutrition (ION)
Blades Court, Deodar Road, London SW15 2NU
Tel 020 8877 9993
Fax 020 8877 9980
Email: info@ion.ac.uk
Website: www.ion.ac.uk

ION exists as an independent educational charity to help you achieve opti-
mum health. ION offers a membership scheme, a magazine, study courses
and consultations

Higher Nature Plc
Burwash Common, East Sussex TN19 7LX
Tel: 0845 330 0012
Fax: 0870 066 4010
Email: sales@higher-nature.co.uk
Website: www.highernature.co.uk

Suppliers of nutritional supplements, they provide a catalogue and free
magazine on request, a nutritional helpline for your queries, and nutrition
consultations by phone or in person

The Nutri Centre
7 Park Crescent, London W1B 1PF
Tel: 020 7436 5122
Fax: 020 7436 5171
Email: enq@nutricentre.com
Website: www.nutricentre.com

Shop at the above address or mail order for a large selection of books and supplements

The Nutritional Cancer Therapy Trust
Skyecroft, Wonham Way, Gomsall, Surrey GU5 9 NZ
Tel: 01636 612707
Email: enquiries@defeatingcancer.co.uk
Website: www.defeatingcancer.co.uk

Information on a therapy that applies conventional science in a naturopathic way, in order to gain remission from cancer and other diseases

Yorktest Laboratories Ltd
Murton Way, Osbaldwick, York YO19 5US
Tel: 0800 074 6185
Fax: 01904 422000
Email: clientsupport@yorktest.com
Website: www.yorktest.com

Provides 'pin prick' blood testing for allergies and food sensitivities and supplies relevant books. Tests are also available at Lloyds and selected Moss pharmacies throughout the UK

Health Screening (UK) Ltd
1 Church Square, Taunton, Somerset TA1 1SA
Tel: 01823 325023
Fax: 01904 422000
Email: sales@healthscreeningltd.co.uk
Website: www.healthscreening.co.uk

Provides details of food sensitivity testers (using vega testing) working in over 700 centres throughout the UK

Index